The Forsythe Anti-Cancer DIET

By

James W Forsythe M.D., H.M.D.

Foreword by Garry Gordon, MD, DO, MD(H)

The Forsythe Anti-Cancer Diet

Century Wellness Publishing

Copyright © 2013, By James W. Forsythe, M.D., H.M.D.

All Rights Reserved, including the right of reproduction in whole
or in part in any form. This is a first edition.

Forsythe, James W., M.D., H.M.D.

Book Design: Patty Atcheson Melton

Cover Photograph: Jeff Dow

1. Health   2. Diets

NOTICE: The author of this book used his best efforts to prepare
this publication. The author and publisher make no representation
or warranties with respect to the accuracy, applicability, or
completeness of the contents of this book. The author disclaims
any warranties (express or implied), as to the merchantability, or
fitness of the text herein for any particular purpose. The author
and publisher shall in no event be held liable for any loss or
other damages, including but not limited to special, incidental,
consequential or other damages due to the printed contents herein.

This book contains material protected under International and
Federal Copyright Laws and Treaties. Any unauthorized reprint or
use of this material is prohibited, under civil and federal
and governmental penalties.

ISBN: 978-0-9848383-6-3

Dedication

To my entire office staff, including my wife, Earlene, an administrator and an Advanced Nurse Practitioner (A.P.N.), office manager Valerie Kilgore, R.N., and my two associates, Dr. Maged Maged, and Dr. Samuel Winter.

In addition, I dedicate this to all my wonderful, inspiring and courageous patients who understand that nutrition and careful dieting are key factors in managing cancer. They know that carrying out the dietary recommendations is absolutely necessary to achieving a full remission and possibly a cure.

Foreword
By
Garry Gordon, MD, DO, MD(H)

Whenever I encounter James W. Forsythe, M.D., H.M.D., I feel admiration for him as a friend and as a medical professional as well. Like Doctor Forsythe and many other homeopaths, I have felt an urgent need to help patients with natural remedies, particularly specific untainted organic foods, herbs and supplements deemed ideal for cancer or other specific ailments. As you might imagine, the general public has yearned for these non-toxic solutions. Yet the mainstream medical industry continues pushing dangerous, ineffective drugs on patients—all while failing to mention or even to give critical advice on the essential needs for specific foods.

Natural approaches to medicine have always been a vital interest to me, especially since I received an honorary M.D. degree from the University of California, Irvine, in 1962, and completed my radiology residency in 1964 from Mt. Zion in San Francisco. Also a former Medical Director for many years at a leading international laboratory for trace mineral analysis, the Mineral Lab in Hayward, California, I have followed with great interest the advancements of Doctor Forsythe's career in recent decades.

Even after serving on the Board of Homeopathic Medical Examiners, I closely followed the many advances in natural medicine remedies that Doctor Forsythe played an integral role in launching. As you might very well imagine, Doctor Forsythe's bold style in pushing for natural health remedies incurred the wrath of mainstream oncologists and also the huge pharmaceutical industry, known as Big Pharma.

Throughout those years, particularly from the 1990s and beyond, the public demand grew multi-fold for the services of experienced homeopaths or for cutting-edge natural medical ventures such as mine, the Gordon Research Institute.

Especially as the 21ˢᵗ Century approached, in operating our separate unaffiliated clinics and medical practices, we each watched with great interest as the standard medicine industry tried to deceive the public into wrongly believing that homeopaths are merely "quacks" whose remedies invariably fail.

Even so, many consumers became suspicious or leery of mainstream doctors, perhaps because standard-medicine physicians often over-prescribed addictive, expensive pain medicines. Compounding problems, as they still do today, in many cases standard allopathic physicians also failed to tell their patients of potentially effective natural remedies.

My professional admiration for Doctor Forsythe grew multi-fold during the 1990s, when he added a homeopathic license to his repertoire. From the 1960s until then, he had been a practicing mainstream medical oncologist. Following pre-designated, mandatory medical protocol set by other oncologists, until also becoming a homeopath in the 1990s, he had prescribed only poisonous chemo and dangerous drugs to his cancer patients.

Mirroring the results of other oncologists practicing nationwide at the time, less than 2 percent of Doctor Forsythe's stage IV cancer patients survived from the beginning of his practice until he eventually "saw the light and added homeopathy" to his services.

Like I had previously done and other homeopaths as well, to his credit Doctor Forsythe recognized that the overall mainstream medical industry had been miserably failing its patients. Perhaps even more importantly, Doctor Forsythe joined other homeopaths in helping to take a leadership role in bringing vital information about the benefits of natural remedies to the general public.

As you might very well imagine, among homeopaths gathering for professional conventions across Nevada and nationwide, Doctor Forsythe earned the distinction as a "maverick physician." Among our peers, he developed an in-your-face reputation for fighting the

"Big Brother" mainstream medical system, while championing effective ways to help inform the public about primary medicine's ineffective protocols.

As the Co-Founder of the American College of Advanced Medicine, I followed Doctor Forsythe's efforts in this regard with great interest.

While also helping to lead these essential efforts, working separately and independently from Doctor Forsythe, I also founded and became president of the International College of Advanced Longevity and also served as a Board Member of the Oxidative Medicine Association. Every step of the way, I became humbled and grateful to learn that Doctor Forsythe had also been telling our homeopathic associates of my many professional success stories and results as well.

Like Doctor Forsythe and other homeopaths have done, I felt a burning and relentless need to help bring the truth about natural remedies to the general public. That's among primary reasons why I eagerly read an early initial manuscript of Doctor Forsythe's critical anti-cancer diet book that you're just starting to review here.

As you'll soon discover in the subsequent chapters, for the most part in crafting this publication Doctor Forsythe has pieced together and concisely explained many of the basic and essential benefits that homeopaths have long known about natural foods, herbs and supplements.

Just as impressive, within the pages herein, he has helped describe these integral and important factors in an easy-to-understand way that only a handful of other books on this urgent subject have come anywhere close to adequately addressing. Meantime, the additional medical advancements that I helped lead drew international acclaim, particularly when media sensation and author Suzanne Somers quoted me extensively in her best-selling 2012 book, "Bombshell: Explosive Medical Secrets that Will Redefine Aging."

Indeed, what I can tell you now without any hesitation

whatsoever, is that all consumers nationwide and around the world for that matter need the critical information within this essential book by Doctor Forsythe. It's time for all homeopaths and patients—including those with cancer—to take a positive stand and to push for more good-health remedies such as those that Doctor Forsythe describes here.

Along the way, as you'll also soon discover, as Doctor Forsythe clearly states from the start, this book is not intended as merely a quickie method of grabbing healthy food recipes—and then hoping that those do the trick in generating good health.

You see, like I have done in my own homeopathic career in interacting with my patients, I have stressed that after receiving a thorough initial medical examination, each patient needs to get dieting suggestions and perhaps natural remedies to address his or her own specific needs.

Especially as an advisor to the American Board of Chelation Therapy, and also as a past instructor and examiner for all chelation physicians, I fully realize the critical need to concentrate on each patient's unique biological challenges—while also addressing the person's specific medical issues, if any.

Mindful of such essential factors, I understand why Doctor Forsythe chose the methodical, medical approach that you'll find in the helpful pages that follow.

I agree with his compelling, in-depth, educational instructional strategy, largely because patients often yearn to know why certain remedies such as healthy foods are recommended for them. As if a proverbial cherry atop a wedding cake, this information also enables patients to understand the underlying causes of their illnesses—particularly cancer. As you'll soon discover, as an overall informational strategy, Doctor Forsythe's explanations for the most part often delve info specific factors that cause cancer such as inflammation and the ingesting of white sugars.

With just as much importance you'll be able to review Doctor Forsythe's many controversial answers to questions such as: Why doesn't the mainstream medical industry want patients to know about the benefits of natural foods? Why do mainstream oncologists push only dangerous drugs while refusing to discuss or to mention healthy foods and other natural remedies? Why do specific bodily organs and functions deteriorate, clearing a pathway for the potential development of cancer? Which specific foods or other natural remedies are likely to address or even reverse such negative physical conditions? And, among many other essential questions that Doctor Forsythe addresses, in what cases are certain chemo drugs deemed ineffective beforehand and how is that done— thereby preventing a patient from having to endure ineffective and debilitating standard-medicine treatments?

Like Doctor Forsythe's clinic does, at my unaffiliated Gordon Research Institute we strive to provide essential solutions for restoring, building and maintaining optimal health. Particularly as we collectively and individually strive to bring superior natural remedies to patients, all homeopaths want to do our best in bringing to patients advanced non-toxic therapies from around the world. Doctor Forsythe and I fully agree, as do all fully licensed and educated homeopaths, that as medical professionals we need to administer, recommend or prescribe only advanced therapies or remedies that are proven effective in scientific studies and clinical applications.

Certainly, as I hope you'll soon discover, the "Forsythe Anti-Cancer Diet" protocol and educational process can help consumers go a long way in addressing these critical goals.

— **Garry Gordon, MD, DO, MD(H)**

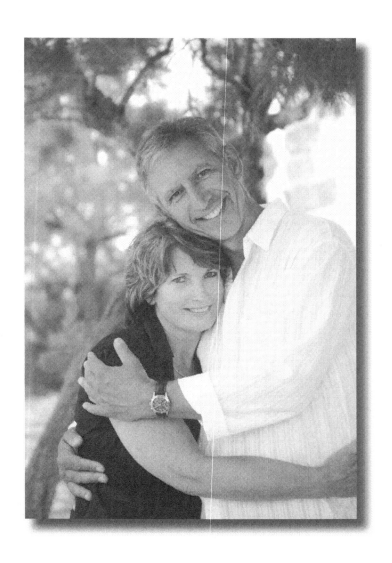

Chapter 1

Introducing the Forsythe Anti-Cancer Diet

Think of healthy cooking as fun and beneficial, rather than considering the preparation of anti-cancer meals as an arduous, cumbersome chore.

The food preparation process doesn't need to be rushed, and with just a bit of pre-planning these simple tasks are usually done with little effort. An added blessing emerges with the realization that as seen in many of the natural anti-cancer recipes found herein, many of the basics can be done up to a few days or even a week beforehand.

Patients who start incorporating these recipes into their lifestyles often begin eating nothing but healthy foods, in some instances for the remainder of their lives.

Although these basic strategies and systems are relatively easy to understand and to implement, some people already used to cooking all of their lives sometimes initially discover a need to adapt their usual cooking habits.

Rather than allowing the food-preparation and cooking process to create stress, you should allow this strategy to take place at a slow or relatively even pace—potentially generating an inner sense of mental solitude.

Improve Survival Rates

At least by some accounts, up to 70 percent of cancers are caused by inadequate diets or eating the "wrong" foods such as meals likely to generate free radicals or carcinogens.

If true, knowing the basics of nutrition, and ultimately embracing such a lifestyle, could easily go a long way to preventing or correcting such disease. At all times particular emphasis should be placed on getting vital nutrients.

To do otherwise is a recipe for cancer, at least judging by a wide variety of disturbing facts about the eating habits of today's average American. Among just some of the most disturbing details:

Sugars: As wild and extreme as this might sound, it's true—the average American ingests more than 150 pounds yearly in refined sugar—labeled by scientists as a major contributor or the primary cause of many cancers. Thus, we're collectively killing ourselves, not just by becoming overweight—but also by feeding cancer the energy that the disease loves and thrives upon.

Obesity: At least one third of all adult Americans are overweight, and this disturbing trend is only worsening, according to the U.S. Centers for Disease Control.

Worsening trend: At least one out of every three Americans are expected to suffer from cancer by age 75, perhaps largely to the disturbing trends involving sugar and obesity.

Stop Your Usual Habits

Everyone interested in maintaining good health, particularly preventing or controlling cancer, needs to start out by doing this one thing—stop.

Yes, take time from all the usual daily worries and routines to put some serious thought into this critical issue. Collectively and in many cases individually we're killing ourselves by either eating the "wrong" foods, or failing to ingest enough healthy selections.

Fully mindful of these essential factors, each of us needs to pay close attention to what we're eating. To do otherwise is to invite disease and ultimately death.

Sadly, at least according to many surveys, a huge percentage of us are literally eating on the run, never bothering to plan or enjoy healthy anti-cancer sit-down meals with our loved ones or families. Instead, lots of people are gobbling "junk food" on the run, much of it unhealthful, particularly harmful cancer-causing meals grabbed on-the-go at drive-up windows.

If you're living this way now, you're sharply increasing the probability of getting extremely serious diseases—particularly cancer—and positioning yourself to die at a far much younger age than Mother Nature would otherwise intend.

People Yearn For an Effective Anti-Cancer Diet

Good, healthy and nutritious food is almost like a foreign object to many consumers worldwide, at least judging from what I've seen and learned from the non-stop streams of patients who visit my clinic daily from around the world.

For many people, particularly those of us within the U.S. culture, encountering good, nutritious and natural food occurs about as frequently as coming into direct contact with Martians. It never happens.

Worsening maters, lots of my patients who incorrectly thought that they had healthy eating habits—even people with critical stage IV cancers—discover far too late that they actually have been eating extremely harmful foods.

This might seem understandable because after all, lots of us in today's modern culture actually are occasionally eating highly dangerous meals.

Instead, consumers would significantly increase their life expectancies merely by ingesting primarily organic, whole and plant-based foods.

Professional Disagreements Erupt

Many standard oncologists worldwide smear my good name, perhaps because the natural remedies that I often use generate a much higher survival rate among people with cancer. A key factor in treating my thousands of cancer patients has been what many of them have begun to call the Forsythe Anti-Cancer Diet.

This unique and controversial strategy which you'll soon find in the pages that follow has motivated many people to change their eating habits for the better.

In many cases, as you'll soon discover some patients who had been on death's doorstep rebounded and fully recovered—perhaps, in part, thanks to my unique diet strategies.

Junk Food Kills Fast

Everything for many of my cancer patients comes down to this vital question: "Would you prefer to eat junk food and die? Or, would you like to enjoy the healthy, easy-to-learn and fun Forsythe Anti-Cancer Diet strategies and live much longer while in relatively good health?"

Naturally, the unanimous answer becomes crystal clear. Right away for the vast majority of these increasingly concerned people the primary follow-up question becomes: "What should I eat to treat or to prevent cancer, how much and when?"

The volume of these understandable and basic queries has swelled to massive levels since I became one of only a handful of integrative medical oncologists in the United States during the 1990s.

As my clinic's stage IV cancer survival rates surged far above the average success rates for standard oncologists worldwide, people with this disease and their relatives have increasingly sought my assistance and advice.

While diet serves as only a portion of the overall cancer treatment and prevention strategy, what we choose to eat or to avoid ingesting plays a critical role in overall recovery and for maintenance of good health.

Power Struggles Emerged

Although jealous standard-medicine doctors strive with much of their political power and financial resources to wreck my reputation, each week cancer patients from across the United States park their vehicles in most spaces of my clinic's parking lot. Some people desperate for effective food strategies and natural remedies drive to my clinic in the heart of the American West, in some instances from as far away as the Deep South, the Midwest and even from the East Coast.

With just as much fervor, patients from across Europe, Africa, Asia, South America and Australia also travel to see me—in some cases spending thousands of dollars for transportation and lodging.

What you're about to discover is why this demand has been so great. You'll soon learn what motivates many of these people.

More than merely desperate to survive or at the very least to recover fully from the disease, the vast majority of these people want the basic details that many standard doctors hope that consumers never know about.

You see, I personally believe with all my heart that if people knew the truths about the Forsythe Anti-Cancer Diet that I'm about to reveal in the pages that follow, the world's overall cancer rates would be far lower than the disturbing statistics that many of us read about today. For the most part, cancer is not only preventable, it's also highly treatable—particularly when my overall diet strategies are employed as part of an overall treatment regimen.

You've Taken an Essential Path

Yes, for less than the price of three or four fast-food hamburgers, after buying this publication within the pages that follow you're about to get lots of the basic essential healthy eating knowledge that many patients have traveled the world to discover.

Right from the start you need to understand and to accept the fact that this eating strategy is not necessarily what people initially think. As you'll soon learn, the overall concept involves far more than merely eating lots of fruits and vegetables. To the contrary, eating far too many of such foods as an overall sector can actually emerge as unhealthy or potentially dangerous, at least for certain patients—so, you'll want to carefully follow the lessons and suggestions described herein.

Fight and Prevent Cancer, Lose Wight and Feel Younger

Almost everyone who has heard the age-old phrase "you are what you eat" gets an unexpected jolt when they learn startling statistics. Every eight-tents of a second, someone in the United States is diagnosed with cancer. Even more startling, every 2.8 seconds cancer kills another American.

This gripping data from the "Cancer Journal for Clinicians" revealed that 1,638,910 American citizens would receive a cancer diagnosis during 2012. The stone-cold forecast showed that

577,190 U.S. citizens would succumb to cancer that year.

From my perspective as an integrative medical oncologist, the primary culprits in igniting these cancers are the foods we eat in the American culture. The danger intensifies due to our contaminated environment loaded with excessive carcinogens, radiation and deadly chemicals.

As a practicing physician since the late 1960s specializing in cancer treatment, I have steadily seen the cancer rate worsen. The spread of dangerous computer components and cell phones boomed along with the decrease in natural meals, foods replaced in favor of synthetic or chemical-laden diets.

Shockingly, the cancer death rate ballooned as the mainstream allopathic medical industry insisted on favoring "unnatural" and lethal medicines or treatments. To help put this startling data into focus, keep in mind that from the 1970s well into the 1990s, I treated many thousands of patients. During that period—before I added natural foods and remedies to my repertoire—the bulk of them died from the ravages of cancer. Back then these individuals' overall medical conditions were worsened by poisonous chemotherapy treatments.

I Discovered Fountain of Youth Miracles

Determined to improve results, during the 1990s I made a drastic evolution in my medical career that sharply increased my patients' overall survival rates.

The first phase of this transition occurred when I also became a doctor of homeopathic medicine specializing partly on natural remedies. In doing so, I joined the ranks of only a handful of integrative medical oncologists in the United States—practicing both "mainstream" standard allopathic medicine as an oncologist and administering natural substances as a homeopath as well.

The second phase of this transformation occurred as I incorporated specific, individualized natural foods and other naturally occurring remedies into my patient therapies, remedies and treatments. I'm pleased to reveal here that as a result, the overall survival rate of my patients increased substantially. Needless to say, my business surged.

In the wake of nearly a dozen health- and cancer-related books that I have authored, the number of patients visiting me blasted into permanent orbit thanks largely to media personality Suzanne Somers' positive mentions of me in her runaway 2009 bestseller "Knockout—Interviews with Doctors who are Curing Cancer."

Capping this off, amid the previous and ongoing successes of my own publications, patients and medical professionals worldwide began asking me to please write what they considered the urgent and vital book that you're reading now.

The Forsythe Anti-Cancer Diet

Responding to consumer demand coupled with the steadily increasing popularity of my meal- and food-selection process, my staff and many patients have gradually started referring to this as "The Forsythe Anti-Cancer Diet." Here are the basics:

Users: The Forsythe Anti-Cancer Diet is ideal for cancer patients, for people who have never suffered from the disease, and for overweight people or those wanting to maintain an ideal weight for life.

Theme: This is by no means touted as a "fad diet," but rather a lifestyle change designed to enable patients to retain or regain good health while reinvigorating vitality and sexiness—referred by some people as "good looks," no matter what their age.

Foods: For the most part these are natural, whole and

unprocessed selections, although recommendations for each patient vary depending on his or her unique medical needs, specific diseases or overall health-related issues.

Detoxification: Since various carcinogens, chemicals and free-radicals are often the underlying culprits in causing cancers and excessive weight gain, the overall health-restoration or maintenance process involves ridding the body of such poisons and of unnatural, manmade invaders into the human body.

Vitamin Supplements: Adding to the firepower, I often supply individual patients with vitamin and mineral supplements designed to address their specific needs. For the most part, this is done to counteract previously ingested chemical-laden foods that have temporarily robbed the body of its essential abilities to absorb vital nutrients.

Forsythe Anti-Cancer Diet Basics

Unlike other popular diets, many of them fads that come and go, the Forsythe Anti-Cancer Diet is individualized to each patient's or consumer's long-term individual needs.

Thus, the process entails far more benefits than a simple "one-size-fits-all diet," such as the Scarsdale Diet, the South Beach Diet and other programs.

Rather than force-feeding our users with a single diet regimen where everyone eats the same foods on a pre-set, pre-timed schedule, Forsythe Anti-Cancer Diet users get unique eating plans.

Each individualized plan is designed to specifically address the person's own unique needs, ranging from addressing cancers or other diseases to levels of being over- or under- the ideal weight for optimizing good health.

Largely for these reasons, the Forsythe Anti-Cancer Diet's alternative approach features numerous specific food selection regimens or schedules—everything designed to address your health issues.

Will This Diet "Cure" My Cancer?

"Cure" is a mighty big and powerful word throughout the medical industry and among consumers. Largely for this reason, seasoned physicians find themselves reluctant to proclaim a patient cured. When such success occurs, many doctors and patients refer to the cancers as "managed," "under control," or no longer posing extreme danger.

All along, no doctor can or ever should guarantee to a patient that his or her cancer will ever be "cured" due to any diets, treatments, medicines or remedies.

As a practicing integrative oncologist and a physician with more than 40 years experience, I'm delighted to report that huge numbers of my patients are benefiting thanks largely to the Forsythe Anti-Cancer Diet being incorporated into their overall treatments.

Every week, I receive "thank-you" messages from many patients who had previously given up hope after receiving medical care elsewhere.

Such kudos bring me great joy, especially after my early medical career. During that period, a vast majority of my patients relied solely on the administering of poisonous chemo—in many cases resulting in death.

Can People Without Cancer Benefit?

A wide variety of patients without cancer can position themselves for potential benefits with the Forsythe Anti-Cancer Diet, even those without the disease.

These range from people with everything from gout to diabetes. Persons who are otherwise healthy although somewhat overweight also seek my assistance.

Anyone wanting to lose weight or to manage cancers through diet should do so only under the supervision of a doctor or other medical professional.

Just as important, you should never attempt to "self-diagnose" yourself or to develop your own meal program based solely on what you'll learn here.

Before launching a Forsythe Anti-Cancer Diet, a patient must undergo a thorough basic medical examination including standard blood tests. Each person's potential success with this meal strategy hinges greatly on results or findings from these initial check-ups.

In addition, we encourage or sometimes require that a patient bring us his or her entire medical file listing previous examinations, results and treatments given by other doctors or health facilities.

One-on-One Care Hails is Essential

Rather than merely relying on medical examinations, at my clinic we also chat extensively with each patient to determine his or her specific symptoms and personal concerns.

What medical issues has the person been experiencing, if any? When or how have specific symptoms worsened, lessened or even disappeared?

Just as essential, we'll need to know your entire personal medical history rather than just recent concerns or problems. Also, what health issues have your ancestors or living relatives experienced?

All these various pieces of the entire puzzle serve as critical or essential elements in my staff's necessary process in designing your individualized meal regimens.

Remember, everything comes down to heredity, your personal lifestyle choices, your current diseases if any and the fact that— through no fault of their own—a vast majority of Americans are ingesting poisonous chemicals or they're being exposed to carcinogens.

Our Diet Serves as an Essential Tool

Many consumers learning these essential details for the first time also should know that some people travel to my clinic primarily to receive treatment for cancer or other ailments. Only after arriving here do some of these patients learn the benefits of the Forsythe Anti-Cancer Diet before deciding to incorporate my system into their lifestyles.

For many patients, this transition emerges during the essential learning process. Using easy-to-understand, simple-to-follow recommendations, my clinic's highly trained and experienced personnel strive to clearly explain what we're striving to achieve, how that occurs and why.

Along the way, many patients report that these simple instructions—including much of the information that you're about to learn here—collectively leaves them enlightened on the critical issue of proper eating. Their minds open up to what for many are "new ways of thinking," primarily my increasingly popular strategy that centers on the fact that natural remedies can and sometimes do prove more effective than standard medicines.

Prior to meeting me or my staff, many patients had been wrongly led to believe by other medical professionals that standard chemotherapies or high-priced drugs were the only viable or potentially helpful treatments.

Yet lots of my patients learn that quite the opposite is true, at least for them. Like all other licensed and certified oncologists, I'm able to prescribe or administer the common standard medicines, drugs or treatments.

The Forsythe Anti-Cancer Diet
Is not Recommended to Everyone

Adding spice to the mix, only qualified patients are recommended for the Forsythe Anti-Cancer Diet while under the monitoring of my clinic staff, after undergoing their initial examinations.

Just because a patient visits my clinic there is no guarantee that he or she will be selected or recommended for a full-scale Forsythe Anti-Cancer Diet regimen.

Even so, for those who ask or who want to receive overall diet recommendations to prevent cancer or to achieve or maintain good health we can accommodate such needs.

From the start, current or prospective patients need to know that my clinic is not a "fat-reduction farm" or a food service facility or restaurant.

Instead, we teach patients easy ways to incorporate their own individualized recommended diets into their lifestyles. Everything from the best or most effective foods to buy to basic recipes gets our full attention on an as-needed basis.

Embrace this Learning Process

Right at this juncture, many readers might expect an extensive list of the foods that everyone should eat, a lengthy list of detailed recipes and a "recovery schedule."

Instead, however, lots of patients tell me they're delighted to discover that for everyone the first phase involves a physical examination followed by a learning process.

You see, as you'll soon discover in the pages that follow, in order for the Forsythe Anti-Cancer Diet to have a chance at giving a patient the greatest possible long-term benefit, the person needs to know how and why specific types of foods positively interact with specific types of cancer. Herein rests the primary reason why the first section of this book covers basics involving good health, plus how my unique treatments interact with the body.

By getting this knowledge from the start, patients have a better understanding of why specific foods are recommended for their personal medical challenges.

These individuals also discover the potential benefits of certain meals or foods, treatment strategies that the standard allopathic medical community wishes that the general public never knew about.

Keep the Information Simple

Adding to the luster, I've designed this simple, easy-to-understand educational process so that almost anyone can comprehend my critical instructions.

Rather than forcing patients to learn terminology that only a medical student or a doctor could understand, the basics that follow are simple enough for even elementary school students to fully grasp.

Then, while delving into vital information on my treatments and the unique challenges that many patients face, you'll discover the essentials of the human body's miraculous immune systems and its healing mechanisms.

As your understanding of these critical processes increases, you'll gradually discover the basic food groups used for attacking specific types of cancers—plus why certain foods emerge as more effective for certain tumors.

Once we've tackled those basics, you'll find information on the various types of foods and anti-cancer diets, most developed by separate doctors, cultures or groups of medical professionals.

Along the way, in order to meet the requests of many of my

long-time patients, we'll delve into critical social and political issues. The many key questions that I tackle range from "how can more people benefit from the Forsythe Anti-Cancer Diet," to "how can consumers convince standard-medicine doctors to acknowledge and to recommend the benefits of certain natural foods for specific cancers?"

Chapter 1 Summary

The Forsythe Anti-Cancer Diet can emerge as a fun and effective strategy in avoiding or treating cancer as part of an overall regimen. There can be no guarantee that any diet will cure or prevent all cancers. As an overall group, the stage IV cancer patients treated at my clinic—including many using Forsythe Anti-Cancer Diet strategies—have a much higher survival rate than people treated by standard oncologists.

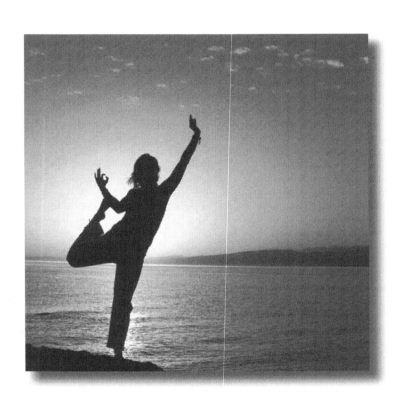

Chapter 2

Enjoy the
Fountain of Youth

Imagine being told that you have inoperable cancer with just one month to live.

Naturally, if you're like many thousands of patients that I've helped, you would find yourself devastated by such a diagnosis.

As I've clearly pointed out in several of my other publications, if any doctor tells you to "get your affairs in order" you should instantly find yourself a new physician.

Yes, there is almost nothing better for many cancer patients than to have a reason to hope. And, I'm happy to say that the Forsythe Anti-Cancer Diet often provides such a motivation.

When touting such benefits, I need to stress of course that results vary and that no two patients enjoy the same outcomes. While some patients receive little or no obvious improvement, many have regained a zest for life as their cancers became controllable.

Thanks largely to the dedication and persistence of my staff, coupled with the commitment of many thankful patients, I have seen and chronicled such positive results many times.

31

Others Gave Up Hope

Much of the time, patients who have enjoyed the greatest benefit emerged as long-term cancer survivors after being told elsewhere that their time on this Earth was limited.

"Doctor Forsythe, I cannot possibly thank you enough," echoes as a typical type of statement that I often hear. "If I had listened to the other doctors without eventually visiting you, I probably would have been dead long ago. And, I'm convinced that the foods you recommended played a significant role in my recovery."

But in at least some instances the Forsythe Anti-Cancer Diet, coupled with other treatments that I or my staff administered or recommend, have played a key role in generating the long-term survivals of numerous patients.

Control Many Types of Cancers

The Forsythe Anti-Cancer Diet has played an integral role in enabling people to regain good health after suffering from many types of cancers perceived as the "worst killers."

Many patients who benefited had suffered from stage IV cancers, listed as the worst level of malignancy immediately before potential death.

Besides pancreatic cancer—deemed by some as the "worst killer"—other vital bodily areas potentially addressed by the Forsythe Anti-Cancer Diet or by variations of anti-cancer diets developed by other medical practitioners include the liver, lungs, brain and prostate.

Much of the time unless a treatment or diet modification is implemented to effectively control or "kill" such cancers, the disease sometimes metastasizes to other organs. Death sometimes results when that happens as cancers destroy the body's essential systems.

Thankfully, I've chronicled many instances where I personally believe that the Forsythe Anti-Cancer Diet and/or variations of other natural-food meal plans developed by others played a vital or critical role in stopping or eliminating such cancers.

Indisputable Positive Results Emerged

For privacy reasons, I'm unable to list specific names and addresses of many of these patients. Yet without any hesitation whatsoever I'm pleased to report that lots of them now enjoy long-term survival.

Using hypothetical examples from a long list of patients, you can consider the following stories of streams of patients who eagerly tell their friends or relatives to visit me.

Among them is Charlie D, a 56-year-old man who had suffered from prostate cancer. When Charlie first visited my clinic, he weighed just 149 pounds. A former marathon runner, he began using a wheelchair within six weeks after receiving his initial cancer diagnosis from a practitioner of standard allopathic medicine.

A strapping, vibrant 5-foot-10-inch-tall building contractor when in his early 50s, Charlie's disease had metastasized to his bones and liver. Before seeing me, doctors in this man's Midwest hometown told him he had less than four months to live.

Now in his late 60s, after regaining his youthful vigor and muscular frame, Charlie enjoys traveling with his wife of 27 years, Charlotte.

"I tell my friends that what happened to me should serve as a lesson for us all, that we should never give up hope," Charlie said. "And just as important from my view, lots of us fail or refuse to realize that we are what we eat—and lots of what we consume in today's fast-paced society contains extremely harmful chemicals."

Successes Became Wide and Varied

Remember that while no results should be considered "typical" including Charlie's, in my mind the positive results consistently became far too powerful and positive to ignore.

Among my many advocates making similar proclamations is the hypothetical Annie S, told by her doctors in Montgomery, Alabama, at age 43 that she suffered from inoperable, fatal stage IV ovarian cancer.

A mother of four children ranging in age from 8 to 19, after receiving this bleak diagnosis Annie helped her already-grieving husband Antoine pick out her burial plot and arrange her funeral. Meeting in private, the director of her favorite church choir agreed to sing "Amazing Grace" at the planned "celebration of life" honoring Annie—whom her doctors proclaimed "with great certainty" would die within two months.

Then, desperately grasping for what she considered as her last whisper of potential hope, Antoine flew his ailing wife to Reno, Nevada, where they visited my clinic. Although convinced at that point that this likely would emerge as their final out-of-town excursion together, the couple chose to put their faith and future into the capable hands of my experienced staff.

An interesting fact here emerges in the knowledge that before visiting my office, the couple had not heard of the Forsythe Anti-Cancer Diet. They chose to make the trip based on positive word-of-mouth about my various other unique treatment methods. Although news of the diet was new to them once they arrived, they latched onto my recommendation right away, coupled with various other treatments that I chose to employ.

Annie Enjoys Excellent Health

Now in her mid-50s, just more than 12 years after she first visited my office, Annie now enjoys vibrant, good health. She regained 27 pounds and retained her muscular but feminine frame, still maintaining her ideal weight.

Sadly, the adjoining burial plots that Annie and Antoine had picked out for each other are now occupied by her parents; a heart attack killed her father at age 78, and her 80-year-old mother died from a cerebral hemorrhage.

On a much more positive note, Annie and Antoine attended the weddings of their son Marcus when he was 26, and of their 23-year-old daughter, Olivia. As if adding a proverbial cherry to the top of these wedding cakes, one year after marrying Marcus, my patient's daughter-in-law, Paula, gave birth to Annie's first grandchild.

"I break out into tears of joy, every time I think of the positive life experiences that the Forsythe Anti-Cancer Diet has enabled me to experience," Annie said.

She re-visited my clinic four times for standard follow-up treatments during the first three years after her initial trek. Since then, she has referred two friends to my clinic. Thomas, who suffered from bladder cancer passed away four months after his initial visit to my office. Annie's other friend, Jennifer, who suffered from stage IV breast cancer, has now been in remission for three years while enjoying a healthy lifestyle.

More Than a "Mere" Diet

In many instances, such successful outcomes result from more than just the Forsythe Anti-Cancer Diet, but a variety of one or more anti-cancer treatments as well.

Like other homeopathic physicians and standard-medicine doctors, my recommended treatments target each patient's specific needs. For a vast majority of cancer patients whose health improves after visiting my clinic, diet modifications usually play an integral role in generating positive results.

In fact, for the most part poor or unwise eating selections usually contributed to, or at least played a key role in, many patients getting cancer in the first place.

Sad but true, for a vast majority of the American and the world population, having huge stomachs or excess belly fat plays a key role in launching cancer.

Whenever you see a middle-aged or mature person who has a huge belly, you should consider that individual a prime candidate to acquire cancer—if they don't have it already. Worsening matters, as just about everyone knows, overweight people have a higher propensity to suffer heart attacks, kidney disease, strokes, diabetes and early deaths.

Positive Results Go Far Beyond Cancer

The many thank-you messages that I receive go far beyond people who had cancer, but also individuals who experienced other health problems exacerbated by negative or unwise food choices.

"Doctor Forsythe, I cannot possibly tell you how grateful I am—your treatments have changed my life around for the better," said Bartholomew W., a 52-year-old drywall company owner who had suffered from chronic kidney disease due to gout.

By eliminating foods containing excessive uric acids from his meals coupled with a steady but moderate exercise program, Bartholomew's kidney problems disappeared within four months of first visiting my clinic. And, he no longer needs dialysis.

While not all patients experience similar positive results for a variety of ailments, many were able to eliminate or at least lessen symptoms that had been caused by various ailments or diseases.

With these potential benefits in mind, you should remember that before my clinic recommends other potential treatments, a key phase of the initial wellness process entails identifying apparent causes of specific health problems. These issues can involve specific foods coupled with the need to eliminate them from the diet, replaced by much healthier meals

.

Helping Patients Discover Problems

Rather than merely eliminating the so-called "bad foods" that the patient has previously preferred, we also add "good meals" that the patient ignored.

That's right, for many cancer patients and those with other health problems, some or all their challenges stem from the fact that they never ate enough of the "right things."

Much of the time this involves far more than merely ignoring the basic food groups that many of us learned about as children—meats, fish, poultry, breads, dairy, fruit, and vegetables.

Among the countless examples too numerous to mention in full is the age-old affliction of scurvy, physical weakness due to a lack of vitamin C primarily derived from fruit.

For many patients such discoveries leave them joyful, glad that they finally found simple, easy-to-implement and inexpensive solutions.

Chapter 2 Summary

Avoid any doctor who tells you that all hope is lost, to get your affairs in order in an advance of a "death sentence" from cancer. Although there is no universal cure for advance stages of this disease, using the Forsythe Anti-Cancer Diet regimen can potentially play a significant role in helping you regain good health. Indisputable, positive results from thousands of my patients suffering from many types of cancers indicate this protocol often helps when used in conjunction with other effective treatments. This diet also sometimes assists in eliminating symptoms from a wide variety of other ailments, ranging from arthritis to kidney stones.

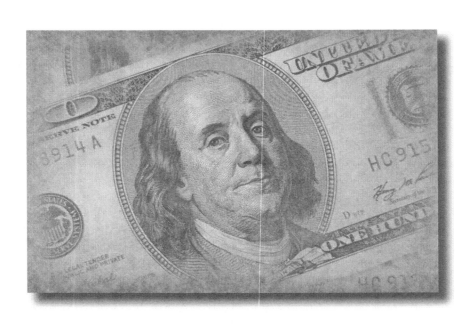

Chapter 3

Greedy Big Pharma Shuns Diet Benefits

Greedy, selfish and profit-oriented major pharmaceutical companies and the mainstream standard medical industry refrain from championing good nutrition to battle cancer. Instead, those entities push expensive drugs—some of questionable effectiveness—and also poisonous chemotherapies, many of them ineffective.

"Many of those companies and standard-medicine doctors value profit more than low-cost and effective methods," I sometimes tell patients. "I've learned through experience that Mother Nature often provides a better, more effective way than what those health companies and physicians are willing to provide."

Such declarations by advocates of the Forsythe Anti-Cancer Diet anger the primary standard medical industry and major drug companies, often collectively nicknamed "Big Pharma."

You see, the huge drug conglomerates are unable to lawfully put patents on effective natural vitamins and supplements, or even enzymes that cost consumers very little—at least when compared to expensive, unnecessary and often-ineffective drugs. In essence,

I tell patients, "Big Pharma is angry because natural substances cannot be patented, and thus those greedy corporations are unable to gouge the public within that realm."

Largely as a result, unscrupulous pharmaceutical companies, standard-medicine doctors and profit-oriented medical facilities including hospitals strive to label the Forsythe Anti-Cancer Diet or other natural anti-cancer diets as "quackery" or even "voodoo science."

My Patients Proved Them Wrong

Blessed with positive results and now with their cancers under control, literally hundreds or perhaps thousands of my patients have proved that my money-hungry, standard-medicine adversaries are often wrong.

Sadly, however, the vast majority of standard oncologists still insist on forcing their stage IV cancer patients to take only deadly chemo and debilitating, extremely dangerous, overly expensive and often-ineffective drugs.

From my personal view, every day the obituary sections in newspapers nationwide are strewn with the brief personal stories of countless cancer patients—many who could have been saved had they known the miraculous benefits of good nutrition.

As far as I can tell, perhaps hundreds of people die unnecessarily every day because their physicians either failed or refused to launch anti-cancer natural food nutrition programs after initial diagnosis. Just as disturbing, many of these same unwitting patients acquired cancer in the first place due to their own poor nutrition habits.

Ultimately, I fear, the mainstream medical industry condemns many patients to lengthy and excruciatingly painful deaths that easily could have been prevented—largely through diet modifications and the administering of certain natural, non-poisonous treatments.

Government Embraces this "Conspiracy"

Pushed by high-paid lobbyists for Big Pharma and the mainstream medical industry, Congress and the federal Food and Drug Administration have essentially jumped into bed with each other. Collectively, they conspire to push costly drugs and poisonous treatments, while portraying inexpensive foods, enzymes and supplements as ineffective.

With huge profits as the overriding motivation, Big Pharma bombards the radio and TV airwaves to advertise super-expensive pharmaceuticals for everything from circulation problems to sleeping pills. Ultimately, consumers suffer from this onslaught because they're never told the truth—that good nutrition and specific foods for each illness often work wonders, in some cases preventing or eliminating the need for drugs.

Just imagine what the airwaves would be like if Homeopathic physicians who advocate natural remedies bombarded the radio and TV ads.

"Eat vitamin C to cure your scurvy, or to prevent or control cancers with antioxidant foods" an ad might say. "We have streams of natural, healthy meals, all powerful enough to help control your specific ailments."

As you might very well guess, the mainstream medical industry likely would saturate the media with a counter campaign—labeling natural food advocates as "quacks."

Chapter 3 Summary

Greedy huge pharmaceutical companies and standard-medicine oncologists insist there is no scientific proof that natural treatments and organic foods prevent and cure cancer. But thousands of my patients over many decades have benefited from the Forsythe Anti-Cancer Diet, which never should be touted as a "cure."

PATIENT NAME:
ADDRESS:

DIRECTIONS:

OOPS !!!
I Forgot to
mention
improving your
DIET

SIGNATURE:

DATE:

Chapter 4

Some "Standard Doctors" Inflict Damage

Sadly, by the time many patients suffering from cancer or other ailments first visit my office their bodies already have been decimated by unnecessary and ineffective poisonous chemotherapy treatments.

A vast majority of these instances involve cases where the patients' initial physicians failed to mention or to address the possibility of refining or improving their diets.

Rather than choosing to point of finger of blame, I realize that a huge majority of these standard-medicine doctors had good intentions or at least followed the rigid, unbendable treatment protocol that they were trained to administer. For the most part, such doctors merely do what they were taught, to give only expensive drugs and poisons.

Additional cases of concern involve individuals who undergo extensive surgeries performed in failed efforts to remove or to obliterate cancer. Yet afterward, even when sometimes told their disease was in "remission," these patients never heard suggestions of lifelong food modification programs—essentially that they had the option to adopt healthier, "less dangerous" diets.

Led to believe they had regained good health, after receiving poisonous treatments from standard allopathic physicians, many of these patients summarily resumed eating the very same foods that likely sparked or fueled their cancers or other health problems. Lacking healthy food habits, much of the time these patients retain or regain their large bellies that essentially serve as "biological ovens that create cancer."

They Arrive in Sickly Conditions

Ravaged by these ill-advised treatments, coupled with their own inadequate or harmful eating habits or preferences, when initially visiting my office many patients are grossly underweight.

Compounding the problems, streams of these individuals lack appetites necessary to gain enough weight to build vital muscle mass and to spark any semblance of overall recovery.

Such physical conditions in turn leave patients weakened, their immune systems compromised. Adding to the danger, due to inadequate nutrition or harmful foods by the time these patients see me they're often left vulnerable to attack from various non-cancerous diseases and ailments, particularly pneumonia—still one of the biggest, most ferocious all-time killers.

For the most part, many or all of these challenges could have been avoided for specific patients. Prior to visiting me, at least some of these people could have prevented their diet-related problems if standard-medicine doctors, clinics or hospitals had guided them toward healthier foods geared to minimize or control specific types of cancer.

So, by the time these patients finally visit my clinic, the process of enabling them to resume good health and regain the weight they had lost has already become a formidable challenge.

Standard Doctors Avoid Symptoms

As a prime example, consider the case of Harold P, a 43-year-old auto-body repair shop owner from Seattle when he first traveled to my Reno clinic.

Listed here as a hypothetical example of a typical patient that I've helped, Harold had suffered from stage IV colon cancer starting at age 41. That's when doctors surgically removed half of Harold's large intestine before declaring him "in remission."

Delighted by this prognosis, Harold promptly regained eight pounds that he had lost primarily due to expected weakness after the operation.

With the blessing and encouragement of his wife, Marlene, a homemaker, almost every evening after dinner Harold enjoyed his favorite treat—a small bowl of white sugar-laden vanilla ice cream topped with rivers of yummy chocolate syrup.

Just one year after Harold's surgery, he suffered from the sudden onset of stage IV stomach cancer. Still in Seattle, two months before his first visit to my clinic, Harold lapsed into a coma and lost 64 pounds amid extensive and toxic, poisonous chemo treatments.

My Clinic Conducts Detective Work

By the time Harold first visited my clinic while accompanied by his loving and devout wife, he told me that they had almost given up hope—but not quite.

You see, jumping the gun from my perspective, Harold's Seattle doctors had told him to "get your affairs in order because you have less than four months to live. There is no reliable cure anywhere for you."

Tearful, Maureen showed me several snapshots of her husband taken a few years earlier, back then appearing robust and super-healthy. That vibrant appearance marked a sharp contrast from the man that I initially saw, emaciated, almost as sickly looking as a Nazi prison camp survivor.

Rather than expressing shock or dismay, I then assessed Harold's overall condition after learning that the Seattle physicians had failed to ask a single question about his diet. Recklessly, those doctors failed to suggest healthy foods during the post-operative phase.

While making no promises whatsoever for a positive outcome, along with the help of my capable staff, I then conducted a full assessment of Harold's diet habits—plus other essential health factors ranging from blood-work results to a review of his medical file.

Refined White Sugar Became a Suspect

Almost as if criminal detectives conducting an intense investigation, the experienced medical professionals on my clinic staff scour through mounds of "evidence." Their hard, efficient work process involves targeting clues or culprits that likely caused cancers.

Thus, proverbial alarm bells sounded when our assessment of Harold's eating habits revealed his penchant for nightly bowls of ice cream. Certainly millions of people enjoy such treats without getting cancer.

Even so, Harold's sweet tooth emerged as a potential primary culprit in igniting his disease. A further assessment revealed his propensity to snack on candy bars and milk shakes.

Keep in mind that when an average person hears of such food selections, they might worry only about getting such relatively common ailments or adverse health conditions as diabetes mellitus or obesity.

Yet many people fail to realize that cancer essentially loves and thrives on—and even needs—sugars in order to survive and to thrive while ravaging the human body. For this reason, I strongly recommend that all my patients refrain from "white sugar" for life— no matter what type of cancer that they have.

Lengthy Lists of Culprits

A lengthy list of potential culprits in sparking cancer emerges. To say any single cause should be blamed for all instances of this dreaded disease would be off track.

When deciding whether to blame "sugar," some physicians and lay people might argue that all fruits, grains and carbohydrates eventually become sugars during the body's digestion process.

Nonetheless, backed up by my clinic staff who gave him similar advice, I strongly urged Harold to immediately stop eating any forms of refined or standard white sugars.

Right away, he began heeding my suggestion while also starting for the first time to enjoy certain specific natural foods recommended for his specific condition.

Within ten days, Harold reported a boost in physical energy, and a loss of craving sugary foods. At my encouragement, Harold thrived following certain enzyme treatments, a detoxification regimen and a diet modification.

Four months later—a full month past the point where Seattle doctors had told Harold he would have been dead—he visited my office for the second time. Then, tests showed his body was in remission from cancer. Now, I'm happy to say all that was six years ago, and now at age 53 this man is thriving physically and doing fine.

Many Patients Got Similar Results

Although a hypothetical case based on specific, documented

real-life instances, the story involving "Harold" is just one of many successes involving Forsythe Anti-Cancer Diet food modification.

When taking these countless successes into consideration, what should patients do?

Should people with cancer depend solely on standard oncologists who insist only on administering dangerous drugs and chemotherapy?

Or, on the flip side, should seeking out and using potential natural remedies and diet modification be considered as well—although mainstream doctors shun such a process?

A vast majority of my patients treated for cancers and other ailments seem to acknowledge or appreciate the "natural" possibilities. So, here is where I come to play, serving both as quarterback and game coach, eager for my patients to catch on and to embrace the easy-to-understand Forsythe Anti-Cancer Diet strategies.

Chapter 4 Summary

Almost all standard allopathic physicians fail to tell cancer patients of the urgent need to have healthy diets to assist in their recovery, particularly amid standard poisonous chemotherapy and radiation treatments. Taking a sharply different approach, my clinic stresses the importance of a healthy, natural diet while also striving to immediately identify and change the patient's unhealthy eating habits. White sugar is often to blame.

Chapter 5

Understand the Overall Strategies

Before learning more basics of the Forsythe Anti-Cancer Diet, you first need to absorb a brief summary of my overall usual process in finding, targeting and attacking cancers.

For the most part, like most physicians I refrain from relying solely on any single treatment method or strategy. Instead, I employ a vast array of techniques, many of them "out of the box" or within a realm that earns me the label of a "maverick doctor."

Without using such terminology when describing my process, Suzanne Somers did an excellent job of summarizing this in her runaway bestselling book, "Knockout."

Hailing me as a "Renaissance man," Somers said that everyone is watching horrible deaths of cancer patients subjected to chemotherapy—making her realize that the "war on cancer is a dismal failure. The 'New York Times' recently said as much."

Responding to her and in full agreement, I noted that a 2004 "Journal of Oncology" retrospective study showed that in a five-year chemotherapy program the survival rate was a dismal 2.1 percent. So, if a person were to undergo such conventional treatments in 2009, only two out of every 100 patients would remain alive in 2014.

By contrast, as I told Somers, our response rate was much better than the 2 percent survival rate for patients receiving only chemotherapy.

"We are averaging 35 percent to 45 percent survivorship, and these are all stage IV cancers," I told Somers. And just as impressive, due to natural low-dose treatments at my clinic, our response rate usually lacked adverse side effects on the body's organ systems—even five years after treatments.

Excellent Diets Prove Essential

Worsening matters, the mainstream medical industry and conventional oncologists that push only deadly chemotherapy never connect the high cancer rates to what we eat, I told Somers.

"You can never underestimate the importance of diet in beating cancer," I told her. "For every cancer, we have a group of supplements that are for prostate, breast, lung, colorectal, ovary and lymphomas that we feel are the most helpful for them. They take that little packet every day, and they have that as the backbone of the basic supply of supplements."

Such overall treatments, and particularly paying attention to patients' diets, marked a sharp contrast from my early oncology career from the late 1960s through the 1980s. The dismal results of administering primarily chemotherapy and dangerous expensive drugs left me somewhat depressed and concerned as the vast majority of my patients died during that period.

In fact, although I followed standard diagnosis and treatment protocols mandated by the mainstream medical industry at the time, finding surviving patients then became extremely difficult— if not impossible—after five or less likely ten years of initially treating them.

Needless to say, this left me discouraged because I had been closely following all required protocols. Meantime, my patients received little or no benefits as I pumped the required toxic chemicals into their bodies. Naturally, this left me thinking, "certainly there must be a much better way than this."

Homeopathy Opened Wonderful Doors

While a licensed and certified standard-medicine oncologist, I noticed the impressive results generated by practitioners of homeopathic medicine in Nevada, where state-mandated boards monitored and regulated their activities.

Magnetized by their results coupled with the high degree of professionalism among such practitioners, I liked the fact that these medical professionals refrained from following the typical protocol of oncologists. Many homeopaths rarely use chemotherapy, or even radiation therapy.

Imagine my reaction upon realizing that as an overall group of physicians, their alternative methods generated better results than my former standard-medicine patients experienced.

Energized and determined to push the envelope within the field of oncology, I made what many other mainstream doctors might have considered a risky or perhaps even "foolish decision." I decided to become a certified, licensed homeopath as well as a conventional oncologist.

If successful in adding natural medicines to my repertoire, I would become one of only a handful of oncologist who dared make such an attempt. Upon receiving my homeopath license, I became determined to administer innovative treatments.

Jealousy Erupted in the Industry

Focused mostly on the almighty dollar rather than primarily

patients' needs, some mainstream oncologists erupted into rages of criticism and distain.

Lots of them started labeling me as a "quack," as my patients' overall rate of long-term survivorship increased markedly. Meantime, the survival results of patients seeing mainstream oncologists remained dismal and pathetic.

Were these jealousies strictly professional? Had I upset the proverbial apple cart, sending shockwaves through the medical industry? And, were the rumors true, that some mainstream doctors flat-out ordered patients to avoid my clinic?

Thick-skinned by this point to such harsh criticisms and putting my patients' needs at the forefront, I pushed forward with my plans to give qualified cancer patients anti-cancer meal plans, vitamins and dietary supplements.

Carefully following my well-researched criteria and protocols, my staff administered many of these beneficial, non-toxic substances both orally and intravenously on specified protocols.

Integrative Medical Oncologist

By taking this proverbial "leap of faith" on behalf of my patients, I became what health professionals call a licensed "integrative medical oncologist."

While creating an effective anti-cancer diet became one of my top priorities, in my new capacity as an integrative doctor I also needed to essentially walk a fine line—traversing a proverbial tightrope to maintain my medical licenses.

Essentially on a professional level, I needed to skillfully traverse a proverbial minefield, to fulfill the requirements of my oncology license in standard medicine and separately to maintain my homeopathic license.

James W. Forsythe, M.D., H.M.D.

In Nevada certain state-mandated requirements imposed
on oncologists prohibit some treatments that homeopaths
can administer. Thus, while determined to develop what
eventually became the Forsythe Anti-Cancer Diet, I created or
refined treatment methods and criteria essential in meeting all
requirements—while keeping the entire process transparent.

As many Silver State medical professionals know, this ignited
the wrath of some standard-medicine doctors within my region,
while others applauded my techniques.

Patients Soon Discovered My Efforts

Determined to avoid physicians who insisted on administering
poisonous chemo, steadily increasing numbers of patients from
around the world began traveling to my clinic. Meantime, starting
in the late 1990s I began fine-tuning the anti-cancer food selection
process.

Throughout this initial phase into the first several years of
this century, I continued to attend the required or recommended
conferences of standard mainstream oncologists. Essential ongoing
education rules also required that I keep up to date with ongoing
developments, medicines, treatments and results within the
industry.

More than ever, the continually dismal results of mainstream
oncology led me to believe that I had made the right decision to
add homeopathy to my medical practice.

You see, in much the same way that they had done in the
1970s through 1990s, mainstream oncologists still recommended
a strict protocol of administering poisonous chemo. Each patient's
individual regimens usually began on Mondays at infusion centers.

For the most part, oncologists who ordered their patients
to follow this deadly routine assured themselves of avoiding

53

any troubles if the treatments killed the patient. All along, any mainstream doctor who dared mention healthy anti-cancer food, dietary supplements or vitamins would become subjected to unwarranted harsh criticism or even banishment by their peers.

Chapter 5 Summary

I steadily began developing the Forsythe Anti-Cancer Diet several decades ago. Much of this initial research was done during the 1970s and 1980s. During that time as a standard-medicine oncologist only 2 percent of my thousands of patients survived from cancer and debilitating high-dose chemotherapy. Determined to find a better way, in the 1990s I added natural medicine to my repertoire, becoming a homeopath. Then my patient survival rate increased markedly, in part I believe due to natural foods that I started recommending. Meals were chosen to meet each patient's individual needs. Many standard physicians in my community became enraged and jealous, striving to discourage patients from heeding my advice. The mainstream medical industry refused to budge, still insisting on using extremely dangerous chemo.

Chapter 6

Protect Patients' Rights

Before a patient starts his or her individualized, personalized Forsythe Anti-Cancer Diet, the person has an essential need to know my clinic's basic treatment process.

Remember, only by first having this important knowledge can the person incorporate my recommended food selections into a predictable and effective lifestyle habit.

To help put this into clear perspective, think of the challenge this way. Before understanding "why" specific foods are avoided or recommended, patients also need to know what, when, where and how everything interacts with their overall treatment—plus who qualifies to receive specific medicines or food recommendations.

Using these basics as the foundation for potential progress, many patients express delight when first learning that paw-paw from Nature's Sunshine is among numerous natural substances that I often recommend, depending on specific chemo-sensitivity results.

This critical substance possessing important affects on the energetics of cancer cells comes from pawpaw trees grown in the Southeast United States.

Poly-MVA Enters the Mix

Immediately upon becoming a homeopath, I became intrigued by a unique and powerful substance called Poly-MVA, a complex of lipoic acid and palladium packed with numerous vitamins.

My curiosity intensified when homeopaths at conferences for that industry began urging me to study this substance, largely credited for putting cancers into five-year remissions and possibly cures.

Even so, at that early juncture there still were no long-term case studies on Poly-MVA that the mainstream medical industry could seriously review. Adding to the challenge, standard oncologists likely would pay no attention to any Poly-MVA treatment case study because the substance contains natural substances rather than Big Pharma chemo-based poisons.

Determined to discover and to accurately chronicle any positive results, I teamed up in a comprehensive study with San Diego Dr. Albert Sanchez, the CEO of Amarc, the main distributor of Poly-MVA. He supplied Poly-MVA for free to 225 of my stage IV cancer patients.

Far surpassing the typical and predictable 2.1 percent response rates of patients treated by standard oncologists, five years after Poly-MVA treatments from 35 percent to 40 percent of my patients had survived.

Diet Became Critical

As these undeniably impressive results emerged, the importance of diet in enabling the overall treatment process to become effective became increasingly critical.

Patients needed to know what to eat and foods to avoid for their own cancers and blood types, plus the best meal and snack selections to interact with treatments.

We found that when patients carefully adhere to my easy-to-follow meal instructions, the vast majority of those who received Poly-MVA lacked adverse side effects five years after treatments. And, continually adhering to their individualized meal programs played an important role in preventing the re-emergence of cancer.

Discover the Forsythe Immune Therapy

Strengthening our anti-cancer weaponry, the Forsythe Immune Therapy mixes with the proper individualized diets and other treatments in giving cancer patients a proverbial upper hand against their disease.

Taken until their tumors go into remission, none of these supplements or the other natural homeopathic treatments generate toxicity within the body. This marks a sharp contrast to poisonous chemo and expensive drugs pushed by standard oncologists.

"Doctor Forsythe, this was so easy—I didn't have to get sick," some patients say. "I didn't become more ill due to treatments; I simply got better. I can't possibly begin to thank you enough."

Dieting During Chemo

Certain specific types of cancer cases coupled with a particular patient's personal medical conditions respond well to low-dose chemo. These cases mandate low-dose insulin therapy, which is non-toxic because we administer levels at only 10 percent to 20 percent of the usual dose.

While low-dose chemo and low-dose insulin might not seem like treatments that could possibly be effective, all this is done to essentially "trick" the cancer. On a casual basis, I like to call this a "smart-bomb" process.

Cancers have certain weaknesses that make this possible. The individual cancer cell surfaces are loaded with insulin receptors. This, in turn, serves as the vulnerability that my intravenous mixtures can attack with low-dose chemo. Amazingly, the PET Scan used to detect cancers utilizes this same principle.

The insulin essentially serves as the proverbial dynamite. The "trick" comes to play when the cancer's vulnerable surface-laden insulin receptors open their pores—fooled into reacting as if a simple sugar is available. This, in turn, makes the cancer more susceptible to destruction by the low-dose chemo.

Once again, following a unique, individualized Forsythe Anti-Cancer Diet regime becomes essential to the patient during this process. The person must maintain overall physical strength made possible by "good" foods, while also eating meals less likely to contribute to adverse side effects or to reignite cancer.

Avoid Sugars at All Costs

Once again, especially at this juncture, patients must remember that to help ensure the effectiveness of such treatments, they need to avoid foods containing white sugars, refined sugars or what lay people call "simple sugars."

In essence, all our cancer patients are put on sugar-free diets, foods and meal selections that lack these characteristics. This food restriction emerges as a critical part of the treatment process, particularly for patients receiving low-dose chemo.

You see, cancer thrives on simple sugars. So, we need to ensure that there is no added sugar in your body during the low-dose chemo regimen.

For some patients this ban on sugar emerges as a formidable challenge, which they almost always meet with grace and unbending dedication. I'm happy to say that the vast majority of cancer patients are eager to follow recommended behaviors and meal selections because they want to get better, eliminate their disease or make it controllable, and to regain good health. In short, they become proactive.

James W. Forsythe, M.D., H.M.D.

Avoid Acidic Foods

As you'll soon learn in much greater detail in subsequent chapters, we also urge patients to avoid acidic foods.

This strategy plays a key role in fighting or warding off cancer because the disease thrives in acidic environments.

Herein emerges the primary reason why I stress the need for most cancer patients to eat lots of alkaline-generating foods at the opposite end of the pH scale from acid-laden meals.

When following this strategy, another key benefit emerges from the fact that for the most part cancers fail to do well—lack to the ability to thrive—in an alkaline environment. Many naturally grown foods are alkaline, such as most primary vegetables. Alkaline water also usually proves effective. Other helpful high-alkaline foods contain or are comprised solely of algae, barley grass, wheatgrass and ryegrass.

By contrast, a huge percentage of processed synthetic meals are acidic, such as chemical-laden foods like hot dogs, certain bacon brands, sugar-laden snacks, ice cream, candy, soft drinks and other foods that have been highly modified.

Cancer Strives to Kill You

The goal of every cancer cell is ultimately to kill you, and thus eventually to result in its own demise upon achieving its treacherous objective. In this respect it is tantamount to a suicide bomber.

Thus adhering to a pre-designated, individualized Forsythe Anti-Cancer Diet regimen becomes critical for each patient's overall treatment regimen.

I cannot possibly stress enough that eating certain foods while avoiding others will make cancer more susceptible to non-toxic treatments. These combined strategies are needed to block or decrease the likelihood of any resurgence of the disease, or even to prevent the onset of cancer altogether.

For thousands of years, the biggest challenge of doctors attempting to kill cancer has been the seemingly insurmountable task of maintaining the body's healthy cells while striving to destroy the specific cells within the disease.

Until the advent of the Forsythe Anti-Cancer Diet, or similar techniques from other lifestyles or natural food-based anti-cancer programs, attempts at treating many stage IV cancers had been dismal in diverse cultures and eras. As natural remedies make many cancer patients increasingly hopeful, word needs to spread regarding the importance of diet in eliminating cancer and in maintaining good health.

Chapter 6 Summary

My clinic uses numerous unique low-dose cancer treatments besides diet that often emerge as effective. A natural, pre-planned diet regimen serves a critical role in helping patients maximize their physical energy during treatments, increasing their probability for a relatively quick recovery. By eliminating white sugars from their diets, some patients assist greatly in enabling one of my unique treatments to "trick" cancers into opening up their biological receptors—clearing the way for low-dose chemo to kill the disease. Patients also need to avoid acidic foods because tumors thrive in acid environments. We'll discover this critical aspect more in Chapter 90.

Chapter 7

Lose or Gain Weight

The average person thinks that the word "diet" means just one thing, trying to lose weight.

In reality, however, this word primarily designates what a living creature regularly eats. Taking this a step further, "diet" can mean what a person already eats on a consistent basis.

On the positive side, just about everyone knows that most people can modify their "diet" or food selections and meal intake to either lose, gain or maintain weight levels—or even to reach or to maintain good overall health.

This, in turn, emerges as essential to remember when taking the Forsythe Anti-Cancer Diet into account. Once again, you need to remember that my diet-recommendation program never attempts to serve as a proverbial one-size-fits-all process, partly because some cancer patients need to maintain or to gain weight. Paradoxically, all anti-cancer diets are weight-loss diets.

Intermix this with the fact that each patient has his or her unique criteria, such as avoiding specific foods due to certain medication or types of cancer. Just as essential, as already stated, some foods are recommended to address specific health issues.

Variety Spices This Diet

When keeping these basic criteria in mind, the entire puzzle can begin to come into clear focus for both my staff and for the patient.

Consider this essential. Tumors addressed by my diet are originally formed in everything from the breast, prostate and lung to the testes, kidneys, thyroid, ovaries and other organs. Additional cancer types range from colorectal cancer and leukemia to melanoma and non-Hodgkin's lymphoma.

With these factors in mind, as one of only a handful of integrative medical oncologists in the United States, I'm capable of recommending specific foods and supplements for each type of cancer through the use of chemo-sensitivity testing. Traditional oncologists lack such techniques.

"Doctor Forsythe, I don't know what I might have eaten without your recommendations," some of my patients say. "When eating the types of meals you picked for me, I never got sick while undergoing treatments—and I gradually felt better."

Medical Treatments Vary

From my perspective, many patients seem to appreciate this specific attention to their individualized personal care and medical treatment needs.

Besides their specific disease-related issues or overall medical problems, I also need to take into account the variations of treatments a patient is receiving.

As a licensed oncologist, I'm required by law to provide a basic "standard of care," always giving cancer patients the option of receiving conventional chemotherapy in cases where their disease merits such treatments. A vast majority of my patients decline standard chemo; only perhaps 5 percent of them elect to have such treatment.

The vast majority of patients visit me in the first place largely because they've already decided to avoid standard chemo. Some of them have learned beforehand of Forsythe Anti-Cancer Diet modifications designed to address their individual needs.

Previous Treatments Dictate Specific Remedies

Once again, I continually deal with the fact that medical procedures performed by other physicians in treating cancers result in serious side effects. These factors increase my motivation to modify a patient's recommended meals.

You see, as stated earlier, some people with cancer look like Holocaust survivors when first visiting my clinic. Extensive and sometimes unnecessary or ineffective and toxic chemo received elsewhere has left their bodies emaciated.

Potential recovery becomes possible for many of these individuals only if they're able to regain weight and revitalize their physical energy. Thus, some of the primary or essential initial Forsythe Anti-Cancer Diet regimen objectives are to:

Stimulate appetite: Administer or prescribe carefully chosen hunger-causing substances such as progesterone elixirs, marijuana or Marinol, a prescription form of THC, cannabis.

Advanced techniques: Some patients have already experienced "burned-out" hormones after treatments elsewhere, and thus their adrenal function becomes insufficient. Many cases involve overly stressed adrenal glands or deficient levels in their bodies of certain essential, natural hormones. I give specific diet recommendations to counteract these conditions. And, as I've told Somers for "Knockout," my anti-cancer diets also work to increase the appetites of some patients after their cancers go into remission.

Other negative side effects: The many potential problems from chemo and radiation range from devastating fatigue and liver failure to renal shutdown, painful neuropathy, severe rashes, lowered blood counts and a wide variety of other extensive problems including chemo-brain. When taking these specific challenges into account, my clinic's staff also considers the impacts on ongoing medical procedures.

Toxicity: Numerous patients experience excessively high levels of toxic substances in their bodies, essentially "leftover" byproducts of anti-cancer treatments or chemo received elsewhere. Sometimes detected by analyzing the patient's hair, platinum often becomes a primary culprit, usually received intravenously. For challenges such as these, usually while administering our own treatments for the patient, certain chelating detoxification procedures and specific foods help rid the body of such poisons.

Varying remedies and treatments: Because each challenge here is specific and unique to each patient's individual needs and problems, any attempt to list the specific foods for every side effect would emerge as a disservice to readers. Remember, patients should never attempt to diagnose themselves; only a licensed medical professional can generate a prognosis and recommend or administer treatments.

Sadly, most traditional oncologists never seek to treat these numerous negative side effects, even the excessive toxicities. Once again, here, we have instances where the foods ingested during an individualized Forsythe Anti-Cancer Diet plan serve vital roles that traditional-medicine doctors never attempt to address.

Chapter 7 Summary

The Forsythe Anti-Cancer Diet regimen features a wide variety of foods. Some patients experience minimal side effects while eating their unique individualized meal plans amid cancer treatments. Some foods are designed to stimulate appetites, while also allowing their hormonal systems to heal or revert to optimal balances within overall bodily functions.

Chapter 8

What Foods During Chemo?

Once again, while the primary focus of this publication focuses on diet selections, in cases involving cancer a need emerges to discuss what foods are best during chemo or radiation treatments. For many of my patients, addressing such matters never becomes a serious issue because of my clinic's unique pre-evaluation process.

When a patient wants low-dose or standard chemo treatments, we first send the person's blood samples to high-tech laboratories in Greece, or Korea, or Germany. There, laboratory experts conduct chemo-sensitivity tests that genetically break down the person's individual cancer cells.

This way we can locate markers that are compatible with your specific tumor, identifying what drugs and supplements are best-suited to fight your disease. We're one of only a handful of clinics nationwide that provide this valuable and highly effective pre-treatment service.

Within this initial diagnosis realm, these diet modifications and treatment choices become possible because the drug-compatibility tests are relatively easy to administer. Remember, the Greek,

Korean and German labs only need to test whole blood. This compares with a handful of genetics-marker testing systems offered elsewhere requiring the analysis of tumor samples that are often difficult to obtain from certain organs or bodily structures such as the colon, brain, liver, lungs or bone. As a result, we can avoid using dangerous surgical procedures.

Of course, at the onset this phase has nothing to do with the person's diet. But doing this procedure helps us modify each person's recommended foods or to eventually assist the individual in avoiding potentially harmful meals. All this becomes possible largely because these tests determine the chemo and drugs that will not work or are likely to emerge as effective in fighting the person's cancer, while also identifying what pharmaceuticals.

Ultimately, at least as it relates to the diet, by taking this vital blood test we're able to indirectly determine:

During treatment: What foods are likely to enable the person to fight his or her specific cancer, or to remain as healthy as possible during chemotherapy regimens.

Non-chemo: When and if the blood tests indicate that chemo would be ineffective, I can modify the person's diet wholly to address the cancer—or to strengthen the body as much as possible during treatments.

Consider the Whole Body

By this point in this vital learning process, many patients have discovered and begun to appreciate for the first time the complexities and effectiveness of the Forsythe Anti-Cancer Diet.

Ultimately, it's all basically quite easy, although the various inter-mingled and co-dependent features of these overall meal plans might seem technical.

In summary, all the patient needs to do is follow the easy-to-understand instructions of my clinic staff's highly trained dieticians, doctors, or nurses at any particular point during treatment, and then afterward for a lifetime.

Among those who enjoyed success by following such a plan has been Alfred W., a retired 68-year-old commercial airline pilot from Sacramento, California, who suffered from stage IV liver cancer.

Before visiting my clinic, Alfred had undergone six months of heavy, continuous chemotherapy treatments near his North-Central California home. Understandably, Alfred looked emaciated by the time I first saw him. Soon afterward, I ordered the Greek laboratory to analyze his blood's genetic markers to determine drugs likely to emerge as effective and also ineffective in treating his cancers.

Within several weeks I received a report showing that two of the three chemo drugs that Alfred had been taking were completely ineffective in treating his disease.

Armed with this essential information, I then modified Alfred's diet to enable him to retain weight and strength. Meantime, I switched him to a drug deemed effective in treating his cancer in tandem with his unique, specific genetic markers.

Now several years later, follow-up examinations show that his liver remains cancer free. I'm convinced that his diet modifications played an essential role in enabling him to resume good health.

Chapter 8 Summary

My clinic uses unique blood tests to determine which chemo might work—if any—for their specific cancers. This process also enables us to pinpoint which supplements are most likely to address the patient's energy and antioxidant needs during treatments.

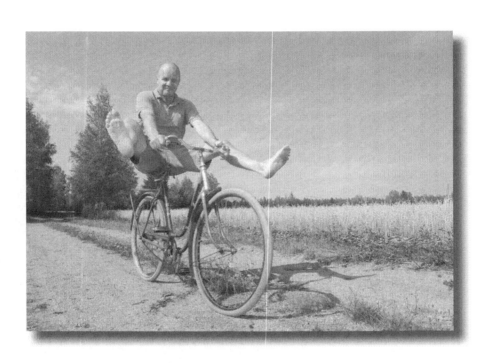

Chapter 9

Take Charge of Your Health

Along with choosing an ideal clinic, medical facility or doctor for treating their own specific needs, desires and goals, cancer patients need to take charge of their own health.

Surely by this point you realize that diet plays an integral aspect within this entire spectrum. This piece of the puzzle becomes so critical that survival could very well hinge on this key factor.

Yet amazingly when attending required or essential gatherings of standard oncologists I read, hear or see very little if anything regarding the dietary needs of patients.

This situation emerges as so uninspiring that I almost want to cry. On the positive side, however, this forces me to admit that standard medicine is failing the very patients that as a profession doctors are sworn as professionals to protect and to help in every effective way possible.

"Dear God, thank you for showing me the way, for giving me a clear, distinct and effective path to help my patients," I often pray. "Give me the courage to do what is right for them, to speak my mind openly on this controversial issue so that more people in need of this vital information might know."

Alternative Medicine Generates Smiles

Gatherings of homeopaths and practitioners of natural medicines generate much more positive feelings. Rather than focusing on poisons and low-survival rates experienced by a vast majority of stage IV cancer patients treated only by standard-medicine doctors, those sessions delve into natural treatments and especially healthy foods.

Certainly streams of mainstream doctors will detest the fact that I proclaim this, but in many regards homeopaths are far ahead of their standard medical industry counterparts in dieting matters.

Everything comes down to the fact that the human body isn't meant to serve as a receptacle and a depository for harmful chemicals, toxins and dangerous drugs.

In keeping with the criteria that Mother Nature had intended, our bodies adapt well to natural, whole and untainted foods. Many of these plants are helpful or at least somewhat effective in warding off, eliminating or preventing cancers.

Mainstream conventional medicine virtually ignores these benefits, while homeopaths incorporate good, natural foods into overall healthy lifestyles.

Pay Close Attention to Food

If I were to give just one bit of advice to cancer patients that I might never meet, it would be "pay extremely close attention to the foods you select and that you avoid."

By now you realize that no patient should diagnose himself or herself, and that only a foolhardy person would haphazardly pick specific foods to address certain cancers. Yes, only a licensed health professional can adequately and reliably address such matters.

With these vital factors clearly understood, I feel a pressing need to give cancer patients general advice regarding food and diet selection.

Cancer patients with medical insurance that requires them to visit only mainstream oncologists should ask those doctors as many questions about food as they can. Much of the time, I suspect, your standard-medicine physician will give vague, generalized answers such as: "Just eat healthy, eat whole wheat, natural grains and lots of fruits and vegetables." Or, as advertised in some infusion centers, "Let them eat chocolates!"

Become Skeptical About Generalized Statements

Any physician who brushes you aside with such condescending statements should cause reason for skepticism. After all, this is your body that they're talking about. This is your potential future.

Refusing to allow doctors to dodge past dieting issues, you need to press for specific, in-depth answers. Every step of the way, keep in mind—especially for those with stage IV cancer—that this is a life-or-death situation.

A doctor who ignores the essential dieting aspect of your overall health is essentially telling you that he or she knows best. In doing so, they're exclaiming: "Simply do as I say. If I thought you needed to know about extensive dieting, then I would have mentioned that or told you what to eat and how much."

Certainly, lots of health professionals are "guilty" of trying to control the communication process—partly in order to manage their work time, and to avoid what they secretly think of as unnecessary, worthless and bothersome chit-chat.

Once again, and I cannot stress this enough, you should remain mindful of such potential avoidance situations and continue to press the diet issue as it relates to your health-improvement regimen.

Waters Get Muddy

However good or bad their own personal intentions might be, some standard allopathic doctors, oncologists or even hospitals and health clinics might seek to refer you to an on-staff or independent registered dietitian.

Licensed dieticians deserve our respect. Such professionals usually must adhere to stringent educational and work requirements before getting certified.

Even so, you also need to keep in mind that the bulk of these professionals lack formal, intensive medical training on cancer, while some lack the necessary complex knowledge of biology. Also, they have no background in homeopathy or naturopathy, and really do not believe dietary habits are important.

To say that dieticians fail to provide adequate or effective guidance would serve as an unnecessary slap in the face to their vital, essential and highly respected profession.

Nonetheless, any stage IV cancer patient seeing such a health expert needs to keep in mind that some of these professionals do not necessary have critical expertise in treating the disease or in choosing foods that effectively interact with a variety of medications.

By contrast, certain dietitians such as a highly trained, specialized independent professional dietitian working as independent contractors with my clinic's staff help develop specific diets for our patients—concentrating on each person's unique needs and challenges.

Insurance Issues Play a Key Role

Compounding these potential problems, a cancer patient's personal health insurance policy might dictate whether he or she can visit a dietitian.

Even more distressing from a medical standpoint, lots of low-level, moderate or even high-end insurance policies fail to cover expenses for patients eager to visit homeopaths.

Adding more stress to this harrowing situation for many patients, the criteria set forth by Obamacare—which I call "Obaminable Care" in my 2012 book by that name—has forced many qualified doctors, homeopaths and dietitians to abandon the medical industry.

"How am I supposed to get well, if I don't know the right foods to eat?" some discouraged patients might end up asking themselves. "How can I determine what foods, if any, are the likely cause of my cancers?"

I suspect that when forced to face this dilemma on their own, some patients become vulnerable to rumors about what food is best. Meantime, worsening matters, some certifiable "quacks" muddy the situation, saying and doing almost anything to promote their business.

Desperate to beat their cancers and to remain alive, far too many cancer patients might be slipping through the cracks—eventually becoming prey to these uneducated, greedy vultures that know little if anything about cancer or intrinsic medical care. As far as I know, no reliable statistics are kept on how many desperate cancer patients "go too far" in seeking so-called cures and miracle supplements and foods that emerge as ineffective when subjected to statistical analysis.

Embrace a "Take Charge" Attitude

Herein emerges an ideal juncture to reiterate the fact that every step of the way you need to take charge of your health—especially diet needs if you have cancer.

"Don't let the doctors dictate to you what has to be done," I told Suzanne. "Seek second opinions."

Above all, while striving to always remain positive, keep diet, supplements and lifestyle behaviors at the forefront of your concerns. Coupled with exercising as much as feasible, strive to minimize or to eliminate behaviors that you know cause stress—such as eating unhealthy foods or potentially carcinogenic meals. (These are described in subsequent chapters.)

Ultimately, the long- and short-term objectives should remain to stabilize your disease to the point the cancer never becomes fatal or causes adverse symptoms.

Chapter 9 Summary

A cancer patient's survival could hinge on diet during treatment. Most standard oncologists never mention or discuss this issue with their patients or among each other at seminars. Many allopathic physicians are likely to scoff at a cancer patient's questioning about the need for natural, untainted foods. However, some medical professions might refer their cancer patients to dietitians. Although their profession deserves respect, numerous dietitians lack intense medical training—particularly regarding cancer. Some dietitians, particularly those lacking direct working relationships with physicians, recommend meal plans that are not specifically designed for a particular patient's necessary treatment needs. Cancer patients need to stress this issue with their doctors, urging the need to work with dietitians knowledgeable on addressing specific issues. If a doctor refuses this request, follow Suzanne Somers' advice and seek second opinions.

Chapter 10

Clean Your Insides and Preserve Your Immune System

Whenever possible under the careful guidance of a licensed medical professional, cancer patients should seek a nutritional approach intermixed with pancreatic enzymes.

My clinic uses or occasionally recommends variations of this technique, first developed in the 1960s by Donald Kelley, whom some people considered an eccentric dentist.

Thanks largely to Doctor Nicholas Gonzalez, this intensive program developed and launched informally by Doctor Kelley was researched, modified and improved to substantially increase cancer survival rates. This highly controversial treatment protocol uses what Gonzalez calls three basic components:

Individualized diet: To specifically address his or her cancer treatment needs, the patient receives one of numerous specific types of eating and food-avoidance regimens.

Huge quantities: The patient receives huge doses of essential enzymes, natural substances and massive amounts of vital vitamins.

Detoxification routines: The individual receives substances or undergoes specific treatments to eliminate poisons, free-radicals and harmful metals from the body.

Pioneers Led the Way

Under the take-charge efforts of Doctor Gonzalez, unbiased research into this sensational technique began nearly 30 years ago. Yet amazingly, the vast majority of the public has never learned of these breakthrough strategies.

The mainstream medical industry largely ignored Gonzalez' findings because—I believe—Big Pharma cannot patent enzymes and natural substances that are critical and necessary for the success of this unique, highly effective dieting system.

Doctor Gonzalez deserves the public's praise and admiration for launching an intense, five-year study into Doctor Kelley's patient charts. Gonzalez did this at the encouragement of Doctor Robert Good, at the time president of Sloan-Kettering.

As noted by Gonzalez' research, the controversial system first developed by the dentist had numerous failures just like almost any medical technique. But Gonzalez found and chronicled many success stories as well.

When developing the overall Forsythe Anti-Cancer Diet regimen, I eventually used some of these critical, monumental and time-proven methods and strategies—but only for certain qualified patients who needed such food regimens.

Success Stories Became Undeniable

During his research several decades ago, Gonzalez spoke with numerous cancer patients of Doctor Kelley. Their remission rates appeared good from 5 to 15 years after their initial diagnosis.

I consider Doctor Gonzalez' findings impressive; my opinions mirror those of many homeopaths. Gonzalez pushed forward with research in internal medicine and cancer immunology, helping to clear the way for critical advancements.

Yet sadly many patients have never heard of these vital cancer-killing or cancer-control strategies. Like Suzanne Somers, I believe that the public becomes skeptical if it has an inkling that a medical advancement was not made by mainstream doctors.

To the contrary, however, I've learned firsthand by adopting these overall basic natural three-pronged diet, enzyme and cleansing strategies that success in treating cancer is not only possible—such positive outcomes can become likely when various factors all come to play at the right time.

Even so, backed by Big Pharma, the mainstream medical industry keeps spending countless billions of dollars on high-paid anti-cancer research, still getting dismal results.

"Regular" Doctors Considered Us Crazy

Although I have never worked with Doctor Gonzalez on a side-by-side basis, so-called mainstream doctors began to consider us each crazy when operating our separate, unaffiliated clinics and medical practices.

From the view of many standard-medicine allopathic physicians, any doctor who dares to suggest that diet plays a key role in causing, eliminating or managing cancer must be a "quack."

While Gonzalez generally followed the initial path set by the dentist, I eventually set my own separate anti-cancer diet regimens with variations for specific patients.

These many natural substances play a necessary role in breaking down foods amid the body's essential digestive functions.

All these factors come to play as urgent and necessary pancreatic enzymes help protect the body with anti-cancer elements within healthy people. The three-pronged diet, enzyme and detoxification system is designed to reignite these factors in people who have temporarily become unhealthy.

Fighting the Goofy Label

The mere notion of detoxifying the body, and also administering large doses of enzymes, certainly strikes many first-time patients as "out of the ordinary."

The three-pronged approach largely hinges on the effectiveness of pancreatic enzymes. Meantime, depending on specific services provided at clinics offering such treatments, the detoxification process can entail everything from liver flushes to certain fast-acting juices and even coffee enemas.

Naturally, patients often get motivated by the fact that many of these natural substances or detoxification supplements offered by homeopaths are far less expensive than Big Pharma drugs and chemo pharmaceuticals.

Remember, mainstream oncologists push many pricy, dangerous Big Pharma products that American consumers and especially cancer patients spend several hundred billions of dollars on yearly.

Taking an opposite route, patients who shun standard radiation and chemo take a courageous stand by insisting on natural treatments.

By fighting for the resumption of their own good health this way, essentially these people are saying, "I have a right to dictate my own treatments, and how my body recovers—as I refuse to use poisons that probably won't work anyway." Ultimately, such patients look to help from me or of other qualified natural medicine professionals.

Success Stories Abound

As reported by Somers in "Knockout," Doctor Gonzalez indicates that 50 percent of stage IV cancer patients who experienced metastases of their disease before visiting him have a "chance of doing real well"—even after never receiving chemo or radiation.

This is extremely significant considering the fact that many published reports and news articles list the long-term overall survival rates of standard-medicine patients suffering from stage IV metastasized cancer as much lower. Some published reports list the 5-year survival rate of such patients getting treatment exclusively from allopathic doctors at about 2.1 percent at most.

Worsening an already sad situation, numerous stage IV patients who receive traditional treatment from standard oncologists go through "hell on earth." Many pass away within four months or so of their initial diagnosis.

By contrast, like Gonzalez' medical facility and program, my separate, unrelated and unaffiliated clinic has helped numerous pancreatic and stage IV cancer patients who now enjoy good health several years after their initial treatments. The vast majority of these patients never have to endure the harsh side effects that standard-medicine usually generates. A balanced, anti-cancer diet often plays a key role in making this possible.

It boggles the mind to face the fact that such results as those generated by my clinic and by Doctor Gonzalez' facility fail to make headline news in the mainstream news media. Regular news outlets at newspapers, TV networks, local television news and radio often rely on Big Pharma advertising. Could this factor inspire those journalists to taint or to refrain from reporting certain significant medical advances, particularly the anti-cancer attributes of certain natural foods?

Benefits of Avoiding Chemo

When chronicling such benefits, I need to stress as a certified oncologist that when a patient seeks standard treatment that person has a right to ask for chemo and radiation.

Meantime, patients who choose to avoid such traditional chemo-oriented procedures might improve the short- and long-term effectiveness of the overall three-pronged Forsythe Anti-Cancer Diet approach.

You see, patients who have become extremely ill, experiencing negative and painful effects from chemo are sometimes unable to eat anything. When that happens the ability to digest foods becomes doubly critical and necessary, perhaps even more so than for healthy people.

On rare instances, my clinic can perform variations of Poly-MVA treatments to ill patients having difficulty in eating. When this happens, striving to enable the person to regain and retain physical energy can become a formidable challenge.

Adding to the difficulty, ignorant or selfish Big Pharma has either failed or refused to develop the critical enzymes into injectable forms. This oversight has in turn made the challenge of treating certain cancer patients with digestion problems even more formidable.

Government Curtails Efforts to Save People

Delving deep into such critical factors, laypeople learning these details for the first time begin to understand that our federal government is literally killing people.

More accurately, the federal government essentially allows people to pass away who could otherwise be cured if the Federal Food and Drug Administrator, and Big Pharma were mandated to assist in the valuable and fruitful field of natural medicine.

These roadblocks occur because high-paid Big Pharma lobbyists pack the FDA and other related federal agencies involved in the medical industry. Pushing this proverbial dagger further into the heart of American consumers, the same mega-corporations' lobbyists also urge Congress to favor big-money firms while ignoring natural medicine.

Needless to say, this leaves many homeopaths frustrated, especially as we commence into the critical phase of initially evaluating stage IV cancer patients and developing each person's unique diet.

Ultimately, my dissatisfaction with the entrenched standard-medicine system here becomes intense. On the positive side, however, my clinic often begins evaluating or serving many patients before they're far too ill to eat and to undergo Forsythe Anti-Cancer Diet regimens. If Big Pharma truly cared, it would develop certain nature-based injectable enzymes likely to help cancer patients. Until that happens, which is unlikely due to the giant corporations' selfish policies, in specific instances where patient conditions warrant, my clinic's staff will continue to administer oral or intravenous vitamin- and mineral-packed supplements and standard natural enzymes.

Chapter 10 Summary

A dentist and a pioneering doctor made significant progress from the mid-1900s through the 1980s in developing individualized anti-cancer diets that enabled patients to "detoxify," ridding their bodies of dangerous toxins. The Forsythe Anti-Cancer Diet employs these methods and other natural systems to enable patients to clear harmful foreign substances from their bodies. Independently operated, independent and unaffiliated clinics operated by me and by Doctor Nicholas Gonzalez have achieved high success rates with cancer patients—while mainstream doctors that have an extremely low cure rate label us as goofy, crazy or "quacks." Unique natural treatments and diets sometimes enable cancer patients to avoid dangerous chemo. But the federal government and mainstream news media either fails to or refuses to acknowledge these significant advancements.

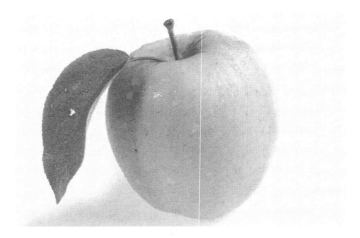

Chapter 11

The Importance of Initial Evaluations

Although the vast majority of patients bring their previous medical files when first visiting my clinic, we still give each individual a thorough initial evaluation.

As mentioned earlier, this process usually includes a complete survey of each person's food preferences, a phase usually overlooked by standard oncologists performing initial check-ups.

This way my staff is able to pinpoint potential "negative" meal- or snack-selection habits. This often enables us to make at least some immediate dieting suggestions.

Another critical aspect emerges when we conduct additional tests, surveys and evaluations that the patient never had elsewhere. Along with a complete blood test, this integral phase often pinpoints likely chemicals or metals that must be removed from the person's body.

This objective often becomes critical. Unless certain poisons, carcinogens, metals and other substances are pushed away, the foods including plants and animal byproducts that Mother Nature developed to nurture our bodies are often unable to achieve their maximum benefit.

Usually my clinic's physicians and nurses have already reviewed many of a patient's medical records before the person arrives. This often clears the way for us to begin administering the three-pronged diet modification, detoxification and enzymes as soon as possible.

Such extra attention to detail often proves essential. Time is of the essence at the point when a patient's cancer reaches the stage IV level. Unless corrective and effective medical procedures are taken at this juncture, when cancer is at an advanced malignant stage the disease solidifies and strengthens its efforts to force the body into its final swan song.

Skillful Homeopaths Serve as War Generals

Military experts tell us that many of history's greatest generals and admirals were exceptionally skillful at tricking or deceiving their enemies. Under such leadership some armies, navies and air forces increase the efficiency and surprise of their sudden attacks.

Well, cancer is "dumb." And, thanks largely to this fact, acting as if a massive army in the "stealth" mode, the detoxification regimen clears the way for vital nutrients from the vitamin-packed supplements to saturate and fortify the body's natural immunities.

Remember, with literally billions of your cells acting and performing together in concert, the essence of your entire body and all organ systems want to live. Rather than receiving and accepting a whole-body "shut down" signal from cancer, the intrinsic, nature-oriented biological systems within our bodies want and desperately crave good nutrition through the proper, ideal foods in order to generate and maintain good health—while effectively fighting cancer.

Simply stated, when eliminating unnecessary and potentially harmful elements from your blood and organ systems, the body often regains its youthful ability to digest and to fully absorb the essential vitamins and minerals necessary to ward off and destroy cancer.

The natural enzymes introduced to your body essentially serve as nuclear bombs in helping to annihilate tumors. From the viewpoint of Homeopaths, none of this would be possible without a solid base of necessary nutrition.

Controversial Hair Tests

Besides the essential complete blood tests already mentioned, sometimes I or members of my clinic staff can recommend a highly controversial hair analysis test.

This aspect of an examination strives to determine highly detailed nutritional information. Many consumers do not realize that besides just examining blood, thorough hair tests also give in-depth information on a patient's current nutrition levels.

Some medical professionals believe that the hair exams do an even better job than blood tests in chronicling nutrition totals within the body. This factor can and often does emerge as essential in developing a patient's overall supplement protocol and diet.

When administered properly, a nutritional blood or hair analysis test can specify a patient's current levels of all essential vitamins and minerals.

Armed with this critical data, the physician has a starting point for developing an overall plan of attack against the cancer— fortified with essential nutrients and effective meal plans.

Use Multiple Weaponry

Virtually all aspects of this early-stage initial testing enables my clinic to establish the specific enzyme types and amounts to administer, a game plan for detoxifying the body and adding nutritional supplements—and also honing the diet.

Remember, much of the time—particularly at my clinic—
the diet aspect is developed by a certified and highly trained
nutritionist. This professional knows the best foods and meal
preparation methods necessary to interact with the patient's
complete enzyme and supplement protocol, coupled with
challenges imposed by the particular type of cancer.

The patient meets with the dietician or a doctor or nurse
on my staff. During that critical session, the person receives an
individualized diet. Just as important, the patient also receives the
supplements and learns what enzymes are required, if any.

Also, during this extremely critical phase, the patient discovers
the importance of filtering potentially harmful substances and
carcinogens from their drinking water.

Much of the time, patients also find a critical aspect deemed
highly necessary for at least some or all of them—how to
eat "organically." For the most part, this usually means raw
unprocessed foods that would spoil or rot unless eaten. (We'll have
more in-depth discussion on organics in subsequent chapters.)

Rather than "boring" as such an overall dieting might initially
sound, for the vast majority of patients this opens up a new world
of culinary delights. And, as you'll soon discover, not all anti-
cancer foods are from crops that would otherwise rot.

Healthy anti-cancer meals mark a sharp contrast to the
pre-disease choices of many cancer patients, whose previous
diets usually consisted primarily of "junk foods" or extremely
unhealthful highly processed microwavable meals and snacks sold
in plastic containers or wrappers.

Remove "Junk" from the Body
Embracing the often-superior methods of natural medicines,
homeopaths treating cancers often strive to eliminate toxins from

vital organs like the liver and gallbladder.

Many of these harmful substances build up in the bodies of modern adult Americans, often because we're collectively ignorant about the benefits of good nutrition.

Methods vary for flushing the body, particularly in dealing with stage IV liver cancer or pancreatic cancer, almost always fatal when treated with standard medicine. For homeopaths the overall objective remains clearing vital bodily systems of toxins, partly to increase the potential effectiveness of a nutrient-rich diet.

Remember, for most chemical- and substance-elimination efforts my clinic offers supplements designed to handle the first several phases of detoxification.

Strategies used more frequently at other natural medicine professionals include juicers and coffee enemas, primarily to clean toxins from the liver.

Benefit from Thorough Cleansing

Imagine if you never made any attempt to clean your house for a half century or even more than 70 years. Surely, the clutter would prevent you from living a healthy lifestyle.

In essence the same thing happens to the body when a person continually eats unhealthy foods over several decades. For many, the challenge worsens even more when they fail to ingest certain foods likely to flush out their systems.

Doctor Gonzalez told Somers for "Knockout" that patients at his office undergo a five-day liver-cleaning flush. His patients take supplements once that's done. For Gonzalez' patients, he told Somers, the standard process works this way:

Start: To emulsify bile and dissolve gallstones, during the first four days patients take a Standard Process product, Phosfood, ingested in apple juice.

Finish: On the fifth and final day, patients complete numerous tasks to relax the bile ducts and liver ducts; the person takes two doses of Epsom salts; for dinner, eats lots of heavy cream intermixed with fruit; and later on an empty stomach right before bed drinks a half cup of olive oil to stimulate gallbladder ducts.

Results: When done properly, Gonzalez says, this process generates vigorous gallbladder contractions. These movements squeeze toxins straight into the intestinal tract from the liver and gallbladder. These wastes leave the body when the person has a bowel movement. Coffee enemas help complete the internal cleansing process.

Coffee in the Diet

Numerous studies in recent years have indicated that drinking coffee might have certain anti-cancer attributes. But coffee drinking can potentially shut down liver function by essentially turning on the body's sympathetic nervous system—which, in turn, essentially shuts down the liver, Gonzalez says.

Conversely, when inserted rectally in the form of an enema, coffee activates specific nerves, triggering the body's parasympathetic systems that cause the liver to relax. This, in turn enables toxins to leave that vital organ.

Ultimately, the entire body benefits because a high-functioning liver promotes and sustains overall good health.

From the view of many Homeopaths, in the long run such cleansing processes clear the way for a potential cancer-free life. This thinking stems partly from the fact that lots of natural-medicine practitioners believe all cancers and serious diseases start in the gut, largely due to poor nutrition or the body's inability to adequately digest and absorb essential vitamins and minerals.

For this reason, the Forsythe Anti-Cancer Diet and all its interrelated treatment processes collectively strive to get the body's entire digestive system into good, fine-tuned working order. So, the long-term process often entails regular cleansing tune-ups. Potential benefits impact all organs within the digestive system, the large and small intestines, stomach, pancreas, gallbladder and liver.

Chapter 11 Summary

Extensive initial medical examinations are necessary for cancer patients visiting my clinic for the first time. My medical staff uses various tests to determine how we can "trick" cancer, clearing the way for various methods of killing the disease and tumors. Our probability of success often hinges on removing carcinogens and various other invaders like plastics and metals from the body. Ingesting certain, specifically recommended raw and unprocessed organic foods sometimes helps in this junk-clearing phase, while also preventing subsequent junk from accumulating.

The initial medical evaluation often is significant in setting an appropriate path toward recovery. Skillful homeopaths use diet and other natural treatments to whip cancer. The Forsythe Anti-Cancer Diet in conjunction with other natural treatments often helps my clinic "trick" cancer into opening up specific receptors, so that low-dose poisons can kill the disease. Removing "junk," carcinogens and white sugars from the body becomes essential for this to work.

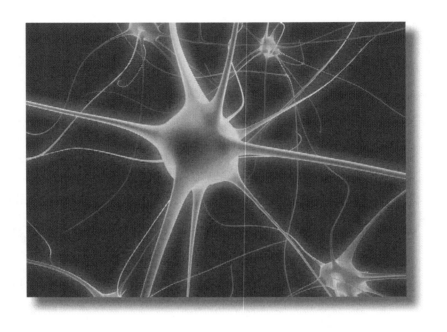

Chapter 12

Strengthen
Autonomic Nerves

A primary objective of the Forsythe Anti-Cancer Diet is to strengthen the autonomic nervous system, with through its various functions ultimately plays a key role in digestion.

Think of the autonomic nervous system as a centralized unit that dictates and controls the functions of various glands and organs. Understandably, a Homeopath's success in regulating these functions can ultimately generate good health by improving the body's ability to efficiently absorb, digest and use essential nutrients.

Besides regulating hormone secretions, the parasympathetic autonomic nervous system regulates the moving and elimination of food and nutrients from the body and liver function—plus when and how enzymes are released and secreted.

Virtually no diet can do much good, unless all functions within the autonomic nervous system work effortlessly like a well-oiled, fine-tuned machine.

Good Digestion Can Help Whip Cancer
Especially when considering long-term results, virtually

no cancer can be conquered or controlled unless the autonomic nervous system's two branches work flawlessly. These are the:

Sympathetic nervous system: This sensational process enables the body to tackle potentially harmful stress. At opportune moments, the sympathetic nervous system diverts blood to the muscles and to your brain. This enables your muscles to act fast if necessary, while sharply boosting the brain's ability to make timely decisions. But herein emerges one critical and potentially debilitating drawback. You see, when optimized to help muscles and the brain, the sympathetic nervous system clicks off the digestive process.

Parasympathetic nervous system: When this system clicks into gear, its various important functions accelerate while we're sleeping. Focused on rebuilding and repairing essential bodily functions, this system targets the digestion system and its related functions. This process rids the liver of bile salts, while increasing the efficiency of digestion. The pancreas performs its magic by secreting enzymes that digest fats, proteins and carbohydrates.

A proper, well-regulated and effective diet enables the sympathetic and parasympathetic nervous systems to achieve a proper balance between each other.

But serious diseases and especially cancers often result when a poor, ineffective or chemical-laden diet puts the sympathetic and parasympathetic systems off balance from each other. These vital internal systems sometimes stop synchronizing correctly, largely due to the prevalence of unhealthy chemicals, free-radicals and carcinogens in today's foods.

Understand Dangers of Unhealthy Foods

According to Gonzalez, the late dentist who pioneered anti-cancer dieting—Doctor Donald Kelley—believed that some individuals suffered from weak parasympathetic systems, while simultaneously benefiting from strong sympathetic systems.

Such individuals were often prone to cancers of the liver, breast, colon, stomach, pancreas, ovaries, uterus, prostate and lungs, Gonzalez says.

Conversely, as chronicled by Somers' "Knockout," he also believes that certain immunological cancers ranging from sarcoma, leukemia, and lymphoma tend to afflict those whose parasympathetic systems are too strong.

Ultimately, the diets we choose can put the sympathetic and parasympathetic systems into healthy balance, or into an unhealthy mode. To enable the body to regain the proper balance, Gonzalez implements these diets for specific situations:

Overly strong sympathetic system: Vitamins and minerals in a vegetarian diet work to decrease the sympathetic process, while increasing the sympathetic system's functions. Large calcium doses tend to work negatively on these patients, who benefit from potassium and magnesium.

Overly strong parasympathetic system: Meat consumption shuts off this system, while increasing the sympathetic process. Unlike people with strong sympathetic systems, these individuals need lots of calcium—while magnesium works negatively, sometimes even causing depression.

Balanced systems: Meats, plants, fruits and vegetables round out the recommended diets of cancer patients who have sympathetic and parasympathetic systems that work together in balance. But for certain individuals, the balance can go off kilter by eating too much of certain foods. For instance, some women with sympathetic tendencies consume way too much calcium, possibly causing breast cancer to start or to reappear. For these individuals, calcium essentially acts as if a poison. Conversely, people with parasympathetic tendencies often have an opposite reaction from calcium, which makes them feel better.

Determine the Type of Balance

Understandably, a key objective often becomes determining whether the patient has sympathetic or parasympathetic tendencies in order to develop the proper diet.

As noted by Doctor Gonzalez, colon cancer sufferers tend to have dominant sympathetic systems. He explains that blood tests, hair tests and even the individual's personality can serve as primary indicators in determining the balance type.

"Sympathetic dominants are going to be very smart, organized, good leaders, good engineers," Gonzalez told Somers. Those with parasympathetic tendencies "don't tend to be disciplined in school or organized, but they can be very creative."

Ultimately, a particular patient's leanings toward sympathetic or parasympathetic or a positive balance between the two plays a critical role in prescribing dietary vitamin and mineral supplements, or in developing meal plans.

Of course, when considering the balance between the sympathetic and parasympathetic systems, any and all potential effectiveness in the treatment of cancer will hinge primarily on the patient's diet.

Make Your Diet a Lifelong Habit

Keenly aware of the need to achieve proper balances within the body, you should always remain aware of the possibility of keeping cancer in check via healthy eating.

Think of diabetes, which can be sufficiently managed continuously amid a healthy lifestyle over a period of many decades through proper diet and medicines.

Based on my patients' consistent overall results over a period of many years, I've come to believe that through diet many cancers can be effectively managed for lengthy periods as well, while lots of such patients enjoy good overall health.

Among prime examples, consider the proverbial case of Monica C, based on a compilation of true stories. When first visiting my clinic 5 years ago, Monica had stage IV pancreatic cancer, and her oncologist told her she had less than three months to live.

Lucky for Monica, when still working with the oncologist from Saint Louis, Missouri, she had refused standard high-dose chemotherapy. Such treatments likely would have never helped this woman, while rapidly worsening her overall health.

Within hours after Monica arrived at my clinic, a mixture of treatments of Poly-MVA and the Fit Protocol was begun, coupled with low-dose chemo and the elimination of all sugars from her diet.

Vibrant Results Emerged

Upon adding insulin to this process, we "tricked" her cancer, and these natural substances then had a clear pathway to effectively complete their jobs as Mother Nature had intended. Within 11 weeks her metastasized cancer went into remission.

Since then Monica has faithfully continued her diet of primarily vegetables and whole grains, since she was deemed has having parasympathetic weaknesses. At my urging she has avoided red meat.

Now more than 5 years later, as shown by tests a tumor remains on Monica's pancreas, but the disease is either scarred over or dead. She's living a vibrant lifestyle with her cancer, which remains under control.

"Just a brief update, I play three or four rounds of golf with my husband every week," Monica said in a recent unexpected follow-up letter to let me know how she was doing. "Doctor Forsythe, thank you for giving me this new lease at life."

Like numerous other patients from my clinic whose cancers remain under control, because she followed the dictates of the overall Forsythe Anti-Cancer Diet regimen, Monica's overall lifestyle mirrors that of a middle-aged diabetic whose disease is effectively managed and fully under control.

Vegetarianism Can Kill Some People

Upon learning that they have cancer, many people summarily decide that "I'm going to become a vegetarian right away."

Lacking a full spectrum of available information, lots of people mistakenly believe that essentially "being a vegetarian is the only way to go."

To the contrary, however, from the information you've just learned, keep in mind that avoiding meats at all times can cause or exacerbate cancers in some people. Remember that meat often emerges as the best anti-cancer food for individuals whose parasympathetic nervous systems are out of whack.

Largely for this reason, I urge all my patients to avoid rushing to the so-called health food stores without first consulting with the professional independent dietitian at my clinic. That medical professional has the patient's prognosis and recommended meal plan.

Once again here we find instances where all patients should carefully consult with medical experts, rather than attempting to diagnose themselves or to generate their own anti-cancer diets. Failure to follow this strategy could prove extremely harmful.

Chapter 12 Summary

Strengthening the body's autonomic nervous system that controls the functions of various organs and glands is among critical objectives of the Forsythe Anti-Cancer Diet. Unhealthy foods often damage the functioning of these critical processes, leading to cancer. Conversely, good digestion can help whip the disease. The long- and short-term goals hinge on generating an ideal balance within the autonomic nervous system's two branches—the sympathetic nervous system, which diverts blood to the muscles and the brain to handle stress; and the parasympathetic nervous system, which handles critical bodily cleansing and repairing functions, particularly while we sleep. Before getting cancer, during treatments for the disease and after the illness goes into remission people everywhere need to develop a lifelong habit of eating healthful foods to keep the autonomic nervous system working well—minimizing any potential impact from the disease. People should avoid becoming vegetarians without first getting a medical examination, because such diets fail to address all types of autonomic nervous system problems.

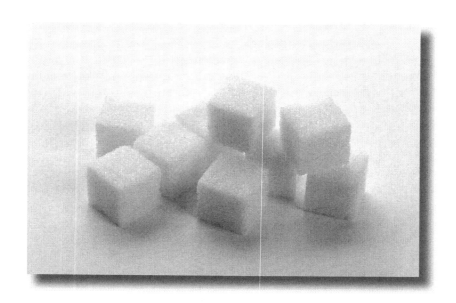

Chapter 13

Avoid
Fatty Liver Disease

A primary objective of an overall Forsythe Anti-Cancer Diet regimen is to enable patients to eliminate, lessen or avoid what's commonly called "fatty liver disease."

These conditions contribute to widespread health problems, extremely slow metabolisms and exacerbate the buildup of cancers. Sugar has emerged as the major culprit in causing fatty liver disease, which can contribute to a dangerous buildup of harmful metals and chemicals in the body.

So-called modern food processing technologies have significantly increased the amounts of simple sugars added to many of the most common foods bought at today's American grocery stores.

This marks a drastic and highly dangerous change from the way Mother Nature had intended. Indeed, not until the mid-20th Century were excessive amounts of simple sugars added to the average American's typical diet.

Food Processing Harms the Liver
Massive quantities of simple sugars added to many of today's

sweet, mass-processed foods have emerged as a poison harming the liver.

You see, in nature typical mammals have never been exposed to such excessive and voluminous quantities of such specific food substances. This poses a significant potential threat to the health of most Americans.

The danger intensifies on a widespread scale because the liver is literally unable to adequately and effectively process excessive amounts of white sugars. Mother Nature never gave this organ a viable and effective strategy to manage these proverbial invaders.

Often unable to decipher how to handle white sugars, especially when they're eaten and digested simultaneously or over extended periods in mass quantities, the liver usually processes these substances into triglycerides—essentially storage fat.

All this means that the liver is given no choice other than to store the sugars in the form of "blood fat." Sadly, this causes countless people—possibly many millions of them—to live and sometimes even to die with fatty, sugar-damaged livers.

Overall Health Suffers

Fatty livers invariably damage the person's overall health. This dangerous factor emerges as bad news, a potential long-term death knell to many people. That's because the liver serves as the body's natural and necessary detoxification center. When healthy, the liver works seemingly non-stop to rid the body of poisonous or potentially harmful substances.

Until recently, the average person associated the condition of "fatty livers" with alcoholics or at least people who engage in excessive alcohol consumption. But white sugar has changed the proverbial playing field, essentially letting more people into this deadly serious game.

People who eat excessive quantities of junk food are essentially playing Russian roulette with their own lives. When a person continually eats excessive amounts of white sugars, sooner or later a proverbial trigger gets pulled. The deadly bullet can suddenly kill the person in many forms, ranging from a heart attack due to excessive weight gain, the onset of malignant cancer, artery clogging, and a wide variety of other diseases.

Livers are Getting Overloaded

The onslaught of carcinogens, metals, radiation and air pollution is clearing a potential pathway for just some of the invaders that have many human livers working on overdrive.

Like the gradual onslaught of white sugar, the vast majority of the many invaders that attack the average liver today never existed in huge quantities a half century ago.

As a result, already stressed by the today's dangerous environmentally harmful substances, today's average liver is already overloaded with toxins. The addition of excessive white sugars worsens an already-serious problem.

Compounding matters, at least based on what I've personally seen, the average American fails to use filters to remove extremely harmful substances from home taps—a primary source of drinking water.

Much of the blame should go to high-paid government lobbyists, who strive to hood-wink the public into believing the average municipal water system is fine. But quite the opposite is true, at least based on numerous independent studies.

Many of the nation's largest municipalities fail to adequately clean or process water. Compounding the problem, most bottled water that's supposedly safe and sold in stores is distributed in plastic containers—endangering consumers, particularly those who drink soda and beer.

Besides polluting the environment, minute quantities of the plastics sometimes leach into store-bought water and eventually into people's bodies. Metals from containers such as aluminum cans can worsen this already-serious problem.

These various environmental contaminants have gotten so bad that, according to numerous studies, the average American's body is loaded with far too many harmful, unnatural, manmade substances.

Follow Basic Necessities

As primary and necessary tools in taking charge of their own health, every person determined to prevent or to eliminate cancer should follow these basic dietary steps:

White sugars: Avoid or seriously limit eating foods that contain white sugar, particularly excessive amounts of candies, ice creams and sweets.

Water filter: Use a filter for your home drinking water taps, or use pitchers that feature replacement filters. Replace or upgrade your water filters on a regular basis, and never trust the statements of public utilities that proclaim "our water is clean."

Fluoride: The primary sources of anti-cavity fluoride for most families are public water systems. So, when using a water filter or buying bottled water, ask your dentist how your children can receive healthy amounts of fluoride to prevent tooth decay. This becomes essential in some communities where studies show that children who drink primarily bottled water get more cavities than kids who use fluoride-filled public utility systems.

Protect Your Liver

The urgent need for everyone to take decisive action to protect their livers becomes clear in "The Whole-Food Guide for Breast Cancer Survivors," by Edward Bauman, M.Ed, and PhD., and Helayne Waldman, M.S., and EdD.

In stressing the "importance of loving your liver," the Guide notes that at three to four pounds it's the body's largest organ. Essential in mastering virtually all bodily functions, the liver works as a non-stop chemical factory.

Did you know that virtually every drop of blood pumped by the heart gets pushed through the liver? This enables the organ to process virtually everything that the body has digested, including chemicals, all nutrients and calories. This process runs smoothly in healthy people.

But when the system goes haywire due to excessive chemicals and unhealthy foods, the potential for cancer increases as the body loses most or all of its ability to process, fight off or block invading organisms or foreign substances. Healthy livers generate a complex enzymatic activity, processing everything that passes through.

"The protective role of the liver makes it an organ of utmost importance," the Guide says. "The organ plays a crucial role in helping the body to break down several essential nutrients, such as vitamin A and D, and the minerals iron and copper. The liver is also the body's mastermind when it comes to detoxifying or getting rid of foreign substances or toxins, whether they come from outside the body (pollutants, plastics, pesticides, and so on) or metabolic byproducts inside it (aggressive estrogens and byproducts from intestinal bacteria).

Understand the Liver's 2-Step Process

Like the guide does for readers, for many years I've explained to certain patients that the liver performs a critical 2-step process.

Without these you would die fast.

The first phase entails what I call a "neutralization" process, where the liver disarms the potential dangers of everything from drugs to unnatural, people-made food additives. A healthy liver that is capable of processing normal or expected levels of such invaders usually handles this critical job right away.

But in order for the entire digestive process to work well in ultimately producing urination and bowel movements, the liver also must efficiently handle the second phase, the processing of water-soluble substances. The key here involves transforming materials that only dissolve in oils or fats but not water into a form that can be excreted in urine or in bile, an internally produced substance that moves toxins to the intestines from the liver.

To make this happen, the bodies of modern humans take whatever route possible to handle the job. This is partly because many of today's modern bodily "invaders" are fairly new substances first introduced into the environment within the past century. Couple this with the fact that evolution has not yet evolved to the point where the human body instinctively or naturally "knows" how to process these substances and the situation becomes critical.

Thus, I fully agree with the Guide when it proclaims that it's vital that "both phases of the detoxification process coordinate and run smoothly."

Healthy Livers Become Increasingly Essential

Respectful and fully mindful of the liver's critical functions, like those who wrote and published the "Guide," I stress to patients that the organ "serves as an essential component" in preventing breast cancer—and, in my view, virtually all other cancers.

Each person possesses a unique liver function process, largely based on genetics passed down from his or her most immediate ancestors—particularly their parents and grandparents. Perhaps this is at least partly why a propensity among certain relatives to suffer from cancer—including of the breast—sometimes runs in families.

While liver difficulties or malfunctions certainly cannot be blamed for fueling or resulting in all cancers, the organ's health or degrees of effectiveness clearly plays a significant role for many patients.

And, largely because of genetic propensities impacting liver function, some individuals ultimately end up with an increased likelihood of eventually getting cancer.

Proper Foods Can Work Wonders

"A well-cared-for liver will function to clear excess estrogens from the body, particularly those that can be carcinogenic," the Guide says. "The more nutritional support you give your liver, the less damage it will take on as it works to keep your body free of carcinogens."

Taking such wise and thoughtful recommendations to heart, a well-rounded and balanced Forsythe Anti-Cancer Diet regimen focuses largely on such special attention to the liver.

As a homeopath, going far beyond what patients hear from standard-medicine oncologists, I sometimes tell my cancer patients that the liver produces what many physicians hail as the "master antioxidant"—a natural substance called glutathione.

As you probably realize by now, virtually every function of our bodies is a "miracle" in performing amazing tasks that we never consciously need to think about.

Glutathione serves as a performance star in almost every regard, particularly within healthy people whose livers function at optimal levels. All this becomes possible when this substance transforms amino acids—commonly known as "proteins"—that we get from foods such as dairy products, meats, fish, poultry and beans. The three types of amino acids that our bodies synthesize glutathione from are glutamate, glycine and cysteine.

Ultimately, the body's immune system can malfunction or liver damage might occur when the body fails to produce adequate amounts of glutathione necessary to process toxic loads caused by infections, chemicals or other bodily invaders like plastics. In addition, stress also can deplete glutathione, because "increased adrenaline suppresses its production," according to the Guide.

Take Vitamin E and Selenium

"Vitamin E and selenium are important precursors to glutathione activity, as well as powerful antioxidants in their own right," the Guide says.

As a physician closely studying and monitoring these nutrients for several decades, I've learned that viable and healthy levels of selenium have been depleted within many crops.

In fact, the Guide acknowledges that "the amount of selenium in soil has steadily declined over the years."

Sadly, posing a potential health risk to individuals whose liver genetics show a propensity for potential cancers, scientists and health professionals have found diminished levels of selenium within many vegetables and fruits.

Compounding this challenge from the perspective of physicians and their patients, according to various medical studies and agricultural reports the degree of selenium found in certain foods seems to fluctuate. Some observers suspect that these variances hinge on where particular crops are grown.

I urge patients to use caution when striving to get adequate amounts of selenium because when taken in large doses toxicity can erupt.

Often available in supplement form under the guidance of a physician or other medical professional, other good sources of selenium include Brazil nuts, mushrooms, asparagus, organic egg yolks, broccoli, seafood, and whole grains derived from non-modified forms of wheat.

Use Foods to Counteract Medications

As a homeopath, I also often go far beyond what standard oncologists can provide—recommending certain foods that can help counter-act the potential dangers of specific medications that are likely to become highly toxic to the liver. Cancer patients should always take precautions against such dangers, especially people undergoing treatments via standard drugs.

You see, many standard-medicine doctors will not say this, but some over-the-counter pain medications such as acetaminophen—a primary ingredient in Tylenol—sometimes curtails vital liver functions. This in turn can lead to highly toxic damage to the organ, potentially worsening the patient's health to extremely critical levels.

As an effective preventative measure, cancer patients on this medication should drink at least 4 ounces of grapefruit juice or eat at least half of such fruit daily. Do this only under the advice and monitoring of trained and experienced health professionals.

A powerful ingredient within grapefruit, phytonutrient naringnin, makes these benefits possible by increasing the effectiveness of certain medications while also slowing specific enzyme activities within the liver.

Determine Your Liver's Health

For all patients wanting to benefit from the Forsythe Anti-Cancer Diet, at the onset—even before recommending specific foods—during the initial health evaluation process I strongly advise getting a basic blood test. Among other things, this enables me to give the person specific data on how well his or her liver cells perform. These essential tests enable my clinic to determine if your liver has previously been damaged by toxins including alcohol or even diseases including cancer.

Although basic blood tests fail to give specifics on how well the liver handles certain detoxification functions, doctors also have an additional exam called a "comprehensive metabolic profile" that can generate such data.

When armed with the data on liver function, my clinic and our dietitian can help determine the best foods, vitamins or supplements to address your liver's specific needs.

As noted by the "Guide" and various other medical publications, B vitamins often play a crucial role in detoxifying the liver. Many healthy whole grains, particularly those not "bio-engineered" or genetically modified by scientists or mega-food production conglomerates, often serve as excellent, healthy sources of B vitamins.

Avoid Chemicals and Unnecessary Food Additives

One of nature's best, most efficient ways to detoxify the liver, removing harmful substances from the organ, involves drinking plenty of untainted water daily while also eating foods that lack unnatural substances. Three supplements are used to detoxify the liver, selenium, milk thistle and alpha liporic acid.

For patients wanting flavor other than water as beverages, good options include teas ranging from green to herbal, mineral broths and a wide variety of fresh fruit juices.

Meantime, patients need to remain just as mindful of drinks to avoid, particularly excessive amounts of sports drinks, alcohol, diet or sugar-filled sodas, and coffee. Drinking some or too much of these "negative" drinks can:

Disease: Damage the liver, increasing the possibility of disease.

Treatments: Lessen the effectiveness of medical treatments for cancer or for specific other ailments such as gout or arthritis.

Progress: Slow or block the progress of your individualized treatment regimen.

Color-coordinate Foods

Another essential and clever way to enhance your liver's overall health and function is to eat only "color-coordinated" foods. Select only natural, unprocessed and non-chemical laden plant-based foods that are purple, orange, green or yellow.

Most of these foods ranging from lemons to broccoli have either anti-oxidant qualities or they lack properties that likely would damage or slow the liver's processes.

Besides the undeniable and powerful benefits of selenium and the amino acids glutamine, cysteine and glycine which we've already mentioned, you should regularly eat foods loaded with healthful, non-excessive amounts of zinc and various antioxidant minerals and vitamins such as A, C and CE.

Perhaps just as important, your liver can benefit from sulfur found in basic foods like cabbage, broccoli and eggs. Ultimately, overall and individually, these foods will work to help ensure that your liver generates the essential substance glutathione.

Herbs Help the Liver

Adding specific herbs to your diet can play an integral role in strengthening liver function, thereby enabling patients to prevent, control or eliminate cancers. Physicians, food aficionados, families and health advocates have known and embraced this strategy in numerous cultures worldwide for hundreds or even thousands of years.

Before trying or sampling herbs, particularly for liver health or for anti-cancer efforts, you should visit a qualified herbalist or health care professional with specific knowledge or experience with such potential remedies. This step can emerge as essential because various herbs or supplements can interact with each other, generating undesired results or potential complications.

Much of the credit has been given to the milk thistle herb, deemed helpful at eliminating or preventing problems within the gallbladder and liver.

The active ingredient of milk thistle, silymarin, has been deemed helpful at preventing cells from accepting toxins with a propensity to fuel or generate cancer. Secondly, as proclaimed by medical professionals, and adding to its own firepower, milk thistle possesses a unique and formidable ability to use its anti-inflammatory and antioxidant properties in enabling the liver to regenerate itself.

As if all these attributes weren't already enough cause for celebration, milk thistle enables the liver to repair its own damaged cells. In some cases, this single benefit alone can emerge as significant in assisting ill patients in putting themselves back on track toward good health.

Collectively and individually, the various benefits of milk thistle work to stall the ability of cancers to thrive, prevent the ability of cancers to move to various organs, and lessen the tendency of cancer to cause inflammation. When and if left unchecked, inflammation can exacerbate the pain of cancers or other diseases like arthritis, thereby worsening overall symptoms and ultimately stalling or preventing recovery.

Various other herbs or food byproducts besides milk thistle that often are credited with helping to improve liver function include orange peels, Oregon grape root, Schisandra, and dandelion.

Strengthen Your Liver-Cleansing Foods

Adding extra firepower to your liver-maintenance food regimen, the "Guide" by Bauman and Waldman lists eight foods credited with helping to clean the liver:

Lemon: As noted by a registered nurse's 2004 newspaper column, drinking lemon squeezed into six ounces of distilled water twice daily stimulates the liver's cleansing process. As noted by the "Guide," although lemon tastes acidic, "it helps raise the pH of your saliva, making it more alkaline. This helps you better absorb the nutrients." Bauman and Waldman recommend that after waking in the morning that you drink the juice from half a lemon within a glass of water. Another option involves mixing olive oil and lemon, a strategy designed to generate a potent liver and a gallbladder flush while patients sleep.

Oranges and tangerines: Like lemons, these contain "limonene," which various studies of animals indicate is effective in thwarting cancer. The "Guide" suggests that these benefits may occur by stimulating the liver's various phases in generating enzymes that detoxify foods or various invaders that enter the body.

Fiber: A wide variety of grains and vegetables comprised of fibrous qualities essentially serve as train cars on a lengthy industrial locomotive, used in hauling away toxins that had been dumped into the intestines during digestion. The wide variety of high-fiber foods includes Brussels sprouts, celery, apples, oat bran, legumes—and certain yummy spices such as turmeric, cinnamon and licorice.

Beets: This plant possesses unique attributes capable of assisting the liver in ways that most other beneficial foods lack the ability to achieve. Beets thin bile, making the liver's job easier at transporting this vital substance to the small intestine. Such benefits can prove formidable, largely because this bile-dumping region serves as the body's primary site for removing wastes— all done after the small intestine breaks down peristalsis and fat. While beets boast these seemingly wondrous benefits, you should buy this food only when organically grown; when produced as a root crop in massive quantities beets sometimes absorb toxins from the soil.

Onions and garlic: A variety of research efforts and written documentation shows that these vegetables possess anti-cancer attributes. Various published reports indicate that the National Cancer Institute (NCI) reaches similar conclusions on the anti-cancer attributes of onions and garlic. In fact, according to a 2010 NCI fact sheet, "Garlic and Cancer Prevention," there are a "host of studies that provide compelling evidence that garlic and its organic allyl sulfur components are effective inhibitors of the cancer process." In fact, according to this document, "these studies reveal that the benefits of garlic are not limited to a specific species, to a particular tissue, or to a specific carcinogen." For instance, throughout many hundreds or thousands of years, garlic has been a key staple of diets within the Mediterranean region, where various studies and medical reports indicate a lower instance of cancer than most other areas of the world.

Chapter 13 Summary

Patients benefiting from the Forsythe Anti-Cancer Diet strive to avoid fatty liver disease, which sometimes generates a bodily environment that creates cancer, blocks the effectiveness of treatments for the illness, and sparks a variety of critical ailments. Fatty liver disease occurs when the organ gets bombarded with toxic overload, forced to process far too many intense concentrations including white sugars than the organ is naturally capable of handling.

Besides excessive alcohol consumption, many of these harmful substances or chemical compounds come from unhealthy folds and even from meals that many consumers mistakenly believe is "good for you." When healthy, the liver performs two critical functions: neutralizing harmful substances to rob them of their dangerous aspects; and processing the materials into water-soluble substances so that they can be safely removed from the body via urination and bowel movements. Good, untainted foods can work wonders in cleaning the liver, enabling the organ to perform at optimal levels—a critical factor when treating cancer patients. Many patients need to take foods or supplements rich in Vitamin E and selenium, each important in assisting the liver. Certain healthy foods also can counteract the potential negative side effects or impacts of medications taken during cancer treatment.

Patients should take blood tests to determine liver function, and strive to avoid chemical additives likely to damage the organ. Homeopaths recommend a variety of herbs or food byproducts to help liver function. These often include herbs or food byproducts that contain milk thistle, including orange peels, orange grape root, and dandelion—plus onions and garlic, beets, fiber, oranges and tangerines.

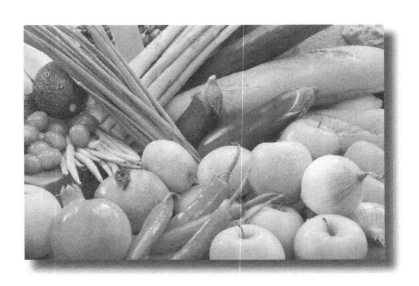

Chapter 14

Food
Means Everything

A frequent saying for thousands of years has been that "a person can have all the financial wealth in the world, but if he doesn't have good health or faith the individual has nothing whatsoever."

Certainly, just about everything significant in your physical life hinges on good health—which impacts your emotional well being as well.

Even more to the point, you should always remember that virtually your entire body is comprised of the food you have eaten. Such factual acceptance, in turn, helps make the foundation of a healthy Forsythe Anti-Cancer Diet easy to understand.

In essence, if you fill your body with nothing but junk food or huge portions of unhealthy meals—that's what you're physically comprised of, litter and refuse.

On the flip side, those who enjoy healthy foods packed with vitamins and nutrition have bodies loaded with everything needed to fight disease and for a healthy lifestyle.

Your Brain Suffers

The potential success of just about every profession and even the potential for fulfillment from personal relationships depends on your brain functioning at peak performance.

Loading this organ with alcohol, narcotics, unnecessary prescription drugs, white sugars and junk food can lead to serious problems in all aspects of your life.

Usually, the "first thing to go" for people who sometimes unknowingly abuse themselves this way is their vibrant health.

Many junk food junkies and even people who consume moderate or small amounts of unhealthy meals, become sluggish and slow-thinking while their bellies bulge or flab envelopes their once-pristine bodies.

The sad fact emerges that many "typical" Americans feed their pets more nutritious meals than they give themselves.

Beware of Inadequate Nutrition

Besides making people more susceptible to cancers, junk food can lead to a wide variety of diseases or health problems in the entire body.

Along with diabetes and osteoporosis, other challenges that "bad or ill-advised" foods are sometimes suspected of causing include arthritis, gout, heartburn, incontinence, kidney stones, gall stones, and many other debilitating conditions.

"I hope it's not too late," some people say when my staff first explains the apparent or possible causes of their afflictions. "If I had only known the dangers, I never would have eaten those bad foods, especially in such huge quantities."

To their credit, I'm pleased to report that the vast majority of patients eagerly and quickly modify their eating habits once they learn that they have cancer.

Certainly, as an integrative medical oncologist I've seen numerous smokers instantly kick the smoking or "bad food" habit upon learning that they have lung cancer or tumors in other bodily areas, likely caused by contaminated or unhealthy food.

Our Government Ignores You

Many people dislike the fact that I proclaim "our federal government does not always work in the best interest of your health."

I feel a responsibility to voice this loud and clear, even though standard-medicine doctors sometimes complain about my statements. As a doctor who often works outside the mainstream of standard medicine, I feel an urgent responsibility to inform you that several federal agencies allow huge agricultural conglomerates to use potentially harmful chemicals when growing and processing foods.

The Environmental Protection Agency, often called the EPA, essentially is following the dictates of high-power lobbyists working for huge agricultural companies. With the blessing of another cumbersome federal bureaucracy, the Food and Drug Administration—or FDA—the EPA plays a significant role in this collusion against you.

As a prime example, as verified by several news reports in late 2012, the EPA cleared the way for a chemical that's also used in sanitizing cleaners to be used in processed foods. While the substance has the scientific name of Didecyl Dimethyl Ammonium, the average person calls this "ammonia."

Brushing aside any legitimate and understandable concern for public health, the EPA officials—encouraged by the multi-billion-dollar agricultural industry—raised the allowable levels of this dangerous substance to 400 parts per million (ppm) from the previous limit of 240 ppm.

Ultimately, most consumers are unknowingly being exposed to and eating highly chemical-laden cleaning chemicals, plus literally hundreds or thousands of other dangerous substances made by corporations.

Contaminate Levels Intensify

The potentially harmful levels of contaminants pumped into America's food supply without the public's knowledge has sharply intensified in recent decades.

In collusion with giant agricultural firms, the EPA and FDA are enabling those companies to make the pursuit of the almighty dollar their primary objective.

Worsening matters on a massive scale, our politicians— particularly those in the White House and throughout Congress— are essentially looking the other way.

It seems that huge campaign contributions and getting re-elected are far more important to our elected leaders than protecting the public's health.

On the surface, everything is done under the guise of making crops easier, more efficient and less expensive to grow. While ignoring the public's safety and long-term health, this process depends on heavy doses of unnatural chemicals. The end result is harmful and even carcinogenic foodstuffs that are easy to process and package for instant eating or quick preparation.

To make this happen, farmers and ultimately food-preparation firms pack our foods with tremendous quantities of harmful, potentially carcinogenic substances.

When scouring the aisles of today's modern grocery stores, most of today's consumers remain unaware that they're essentially traversing a proverbial mine field. The food-contamination problem has gotten so bad that these unnatural substances are a major cause of sharp increases in cancer rates since the mid-1900s.

Avoid Harmful Salts

Further increasing the potential dangers to your health, the food-processing regimen often entails using excessive amounts of salts for storage or for creating "quickie meals."

This sharp increase in salts, commonly referred to by many physicians and consumers as "sodium," can sharply increase blood pressure.

The number of crippling or fatal strokes has increased markedly in recent decades, along with many other ailments stemming from sodium-rich diets.

As if all this weren't already enough to spark widespread concern, fast-food restaurants and convenience stores sharply increase per-serving calorie counts. Much of this becomes possible due to excessive amounts of white sugars and sodium.

All this leads little reason to guess why the nationwide rate of childhood obesity keeps skyrocketing with virtually no end in sight. Shockingly, if this trend continues I fear that the worldwide rate of cancer, obesity, diabetes and other diseases will soar throughout the 21st Century.

While those of us reared in the 1900s got excessive exposure to harmful foods as well, the bulk of those in critical danger will emerge as the "millennials" or "Generation Y," particularly Americans born during or after the 1980s. Most of their parents were baby boomers whose childhood diets consisted of more natural foods that had much less chemicals and processing than typically found today.

Bio-Engineering Dangers Emerged

The government-sanctioned attack on the diets of typical Americans intensified when huge agriculture conglomerates began bio-engineering foods.

This entails using techniques developed during the past few decades to change or drastically modify the internal biology of crops such as corn. The farm companies' goals are to grow crops as quickly and as cheaply as possible.

For this to happen, scientists needed to create all-new synthetic crops, pushing aside any need to protect the public's safety.

With money as their primary goal, the developers and proponents of bioengineering spew dangerous propaganda intended to confuse many consumers. Such advocates insist that biotechnology generates or makes "useful products" for medicine, food or to improve the efficiency of the agricultural process.

Yet as an experienced doctor who has seen a sharp rise in cancers in recent decades, I worry that perhaps—although their intentions might seem good—such scientists might be overzealous in modifying foods, thereby endangering public health.

People Keep Toying With Biology

Standard-medicine doctors and homeopaths need to face the grim fact that biotechnology—and its related scientific field of "bioengineering"—are toying with the essential atomic-level building blocks of plants and crops.

Using highly technical processes, huge corporations are modifying the basic properties of plants that Mother Nature took literally billions of years to develop. Such wide-scale efforts are being done largely under the auspices of greatly improving agricultural efficiencies in order to feed the world's burgeoning populations.

I'm among medical professionals who fear that at least in some cases these processes are generating harmful "unnatural" or "freak" foods. From my view, potential problems surface because the "gut" of the human body is unequipped to efficiently process bioengineered foods—in everything from the stomach to the liver, gallbladder, pancreas and intestines.

Many huge corporations that develop and distribute bioengineered foods proclaim that their products are natural, healthy and good. While more long-term independent studies need to be done, some observers fear that far more harm than good has resulted from the bioengineering and biotechnology processes—particularly the formation of cancer.

Chapter 14 Summary

Food plays a critical and penultimate role in your overall health. Besides the danger of starvation, organ malfunctions occurs within people who have insufficient diets. Brain function sometimes degrades when this happens, worsening the person's overall quality of life. Despite the urgency of these factors, the inept and corrupt federal government does a dismal job at ensuring that supermarkets sell only healthy, nutritious foods. The situation worsens when federal agencies allow Big Food producers and distributors to spray crops with dangerous cancer-causing chemicals or to cram meals with unnatural additives and preservatives during the processing phase. Excessive salts needlessly added to many food products worsen the dangers. The overall dangers intensify because the government also allows Big Food to create unnatural bio-engineered carcinogenic foods that the human body is unable to efficiently process.

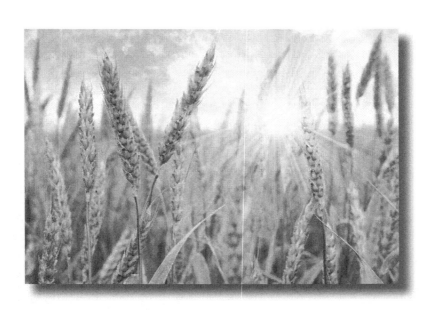

Chapter 15

Wheat
Identified As Major Culprit

A runaway bestseller in 2011 and 2012, the still-popular book "Wheat Belly ~ Lose the Wheat, Lose the Weight, and Find Your Way Back to Good Health" played a critical role in bringing the food-alteration issue to the public forefront.

The author, a widely renowned cardiologist, Doctor William Davis, chronicles his findings that the massive public consumption of modified wheat products has caused widespread obesity and severe health problems.

Davis argues that until the mid-1900s farmers worldwide grew only a handful of natural varieties of wheat that the human body easily processed. At the time, Davis says, average wheat crops grew as "fields of grain" reaching from 4 ½ feet to 6 feet tall.

But since then scientists have developed literally tens of thousand of wheat varieties, the vast majority growing only about 18 inches in height and lacking the valuable nutrition of their natural predecessors. Davis insists that while the original forms of wheat have become nearly extinct, the new species are unnatural and extremely difficult for the body to process. The situation has become so bad, he says, that today's wheat has so many highly complex sugars that eating a single slice of wheat bread possesses far more sugars than a single candy bar.

Adding shock and concern, various medical reports cited by Davis consistently show that blood sugar levels skyrocket to extremely dangerous levels shortly after eating wheat.

Worsening this wide-scale problem multi-fold, many hundreds or thousands of food products sold in grocery stores are loaded with wheat used as filler. As a result, Davis argues, the vast majority of today's American consumers are unaware that they're eating highly dangerous modified foods destined to give them huge bellies. From the view of homeopaths, such attributes become strong indicators of current or future cancers.

Serious Cases Intensify

As both an oncologist and as a homeopath, findings such as those by Davis increase my level of concern for the public health. You see, as stated in earlier, huge fat bellies are a significant contributing factor in generating cancers.

Although Davis' book does not delve deeply into tumors, he describes a wide variety of serious health issues—especially severe digestion problems and an inability to lose weight, caused by ingesting wheat.

Davis describes numerous specific cases where his patients failed to lose weight despite their highly dedicated, rigorous exercise routines and diet regimes. In many cases that this doctor chronicles, the excess weight of these patients instantly started melting away as soon as they stopped eating bread, flour-based products and carefully read food labels in order to avoid foods that contained hidden wheat used as filler.

As described in "Wheat Belly," potentially dangerous wheat-based fillers are hidden in everything from certain ice cream brands to sauces and microwavable meals.

Compounding the problem, the increased efficiencies that refined wheat products give to food processors enable those companies to cheaply make everything from frozen pizzas to calorie-packed frozen lasagna. Financially strapped in a challenging economy, many families buy these cheap pizzas and frozen processed foods by the cartload.

Almost as if stabbing proverbial daggers deep into their own stomachs, many of these same consumers also are somewhat addicted to the sugars jammed within the convoluted wheat products.

Could this be why we seem to see increasing numbers of heavy people in most American families? Continuously disturbing news reports in recent years quote health experts as predicting that the total percentage of obese Americans will continue to swell for several more decades. Although more people seem far more health conscious than ever before, perhaps a vast majority of them are eating extremely harmful foods.

Gluten Intolerance Worsens Problems

Compounding these difficulties multi-fold, by some estimates more than 1 million Americans are "gluten intolerant." Due to what many researchers label as intestinal problems caused by hereditary problems, these individuals lack the ability to absorb necessary nutrients when they eat wheat products loaded with gluten.

The vast majority of these people never know they have such intolerance, which technically is an inherited physical condition rather than a "disease." Of course, entire books have been written on the gluten intolerance issue, and that's certainly not the overall objective of the Forsythe Anti-Cancer Diet.

Suffice it to say, though, that according to Doctor Davis people with gluten intolerance comprise only an extremely small percentage of individuals who suffer from wheat-related health issues.

Besides excessive weight, many people—perhaps tens of millions by some accounts—suffer from severe digestive problems immediately after eating wheat, much of it hidden in foods without the consumer's knowledge. Everything from severe belching to apparent heartburn and stomach acid reflux sometimes erupts.

A vast majority of people suffering from these specific issues lose such symptoms within a few days of removing wheat from their diets, according to Davis. For many people, lots of whom never suffer from apparent digestion problems, the weight loss emerges as the best benefit from wheat-elimination difficulties.

The Pounds Melt Away

Many people report that they initially lose 10 pounds or more within the fist several weeks of ending the wheat habit. For the vast majority of such patients, Davis says, the weight reduction becomes a long-term process, sometimes lasting a year or more for some patients who had been from 50 to 100 pounds overweight or even more.

Following an initial sharp drop-off in weight, lots of these people report that they continued to lose from as little as 2 pounds to 4 pounds per month, for months later.

At least from Davis' view, lots of these successful weight-loss efforts became possible among his patients who still refused to exercise to lose pounds—even after starting to avoid wheat.

Just as impressive, from Davis' view, significant percentages of his patients stopped suffering from specific health issues.

The disappearance of adverse symptoms like gout,

indigestion, kidney stones and gallbladder problems sometimes leads to significant improvements to overall health. This, in turn, often enables patients to resume physical activities that excessive weight and digestion problems had prevented them from enjoying. These physical activities range from playing golf to going for walks, or even so-called "normal" personal chores like grocery or mall shopping.

Apparent Benefits Seem Likely

As an integrative medical oncologist, my initial reaction upon learning of Davis' "Wheat Belly" diet was positive. Yet as a doctor, I realize that much more extensive research needs to be done before the overall medical industry can generate at least some uniformity, an overall agreement on this critical issue.

Also, as to whether wheat-elimination might play a significant and irrefutable role in preventing, eliminating or controlling cancer, additional studies need to be done as well.

Meantime, the "wheat belly" diet regimen seems to have definite benefits, at least from the view of the growing numbers of its proponents. All along, as Davis keenly points out, a paradoxical situation erupts when acknowledging and appreciating his diet regimen's benefits.

You see, a vast majority of wellness and dieting programs strongly recommend adding whole grains—particularly wheat products—to a healthy eating regimen. We're told by most standard-medicine doctors and even many homeopaths that wheat breads play a critical and necessary role in any cancer-prevention, heart-healthy or weight loss regimen.

Certainly, all these factors collectively emerge as a proverbial double-edge sword. Advocates of wheat-elimination argue that avoiding that food is critical, while world-famous organizations like the American Heart Association strongly urge the consumption of such whole-grain fibers.

Wheat Gained a Bad Reputation

The reputation of wheat took a sharp nose-dive during the summer of 2012, when the controversial conservative political TV commentator Bill O'Reilly recommended "Wheat Belly" during his top-rated Fox News politics-oriented program "The O'Reilly Factor." By recommending the diet, O'Reilly made one of his infrequent forays into the non-political realm.

Among consumers who describe themselves as "lucky" for watching that particular episode was Patricia "Patty" M, the 65-year-old operator of an independent graphic design firm that has done occasional work for my clinic and designs for my various books.

During the six months immediately before that O'Reilly episode, Patty had been in extremely poor health. Physicians diagnosed her as anemic, her illness so severe that she was unable to walk up the stairs of her two-level home or halfway across a room. Over the previous decade, Patty had gained nearly 40 pounds, which she had been unable to lose despite her dedicated, unbendable four-day-per-week morning swimming and exercise routine.

For several years, her overall health issues intensified, suffering from almost daily severe indigestion and steadily increasing physical weakness. Patty's overall health issues became so bad that in January 2012 she had no choice other than to stop her regular exercise routine.

Eager for improvement, she began taking natural herbs that only helped intermittently. Meantime, as Patty's anemia worsened, standard-medicine doctors concluded that her body showed no signs of gluten intolerance. And results of a colonoscopy showed no sign of cancer or pre-cancerous polyps. The cause of her slight inflammation of the lower intestine, coupled with her body's apparent inability to absorb or retain adequate levels of iron remained a mystery.

Avoiding Wheat Changed Everything

Following O'Reilly's recommendation although he lacks professional medical credentials, Patty immediately purchased an instant, downloadable eBook version of "Wheat Belly."

Within 48 hours after starting that diet, all of Patty's various adverse digestive problems including indigestion and heartburn disappeared. While continuing her daily intake of iron pills, her overall physical energy steadily increased.

Literally with no effort whatsoever, Patty lost just less than 10 pounds during the first three weeks. Mirroring the results of many other wheat-elimination patients, Patty's degree of weight loss slowed to a few pounds monthly.

Encouraged by Patty's marked physical improvements, her husband, Wayne, took her to Hawaii for several days in September, two months after her Wheat Belly diet began. There, together they walked several miles along a beach in Kiluha, the same community where I had lived with my young family as an Army medical officer during the Vietnam War in the mid-1960s.

"Everywhere we go, people keep telling Patty how great she looks, far better than she has in many years," said her husband, a book publication advisor. "I'm certainly not a doctor and lack medical training, but everything seems to point to the fact that eliminating wheat must have played a role in her significant recovery."

Since starting and maintaining her no-wheat diet, Patty has

suffered from three episodes of digestive problems. In each of those instances, the severe belching, indigestion and heartburn occurred while eating in restaurants—instances where "non-bread" foods contained hidden amounts of wheat used as filler. As a result, Patty has learned to ask waiters and waitresses, "Does this item contain wheat or flour?" But she learned that making such inquiries does not always work. In one instance the food server was wrong, replying, "No," before Patty summarily ate the meal and became temporarily ill.

Whole Body Process

As suggestions increase for more study on the viability and effectiveness of "wheat elimination" diets, unless I or my staff recommend otherwise, the vast majority of my patients still have the option of eating wheat-based foods or flours derived from wheat.

All along, however, especially until more comprehensive studies are completed on the wheat-elimination issue, certain patients might choose to avoid such foods.

I'm eager to see if more research is done on what impact—if any—the elimination of wheat might have on cancer. All these factors are coupled with the fact that blood-work or diagnosis might indicate certain patients are gluten intolerant.

Largely for these reasons, the overall Forsythe Anti-Cancer Diet regimen can include certain alternatives to gluten-packed grains such as wheat.

Perhaps the most significant grains within this category include: amaranth, loaded with greater calcium levels than milk; brown rice, packed with powerful nutrients; corn flour or other non-glutinous flours, often an effective wheat substitute, particularly when making cornbread or corn pancakes; millet, an effective wheat substitute that many people consider tasty; potato flour, which you should never confuse with a common thickening agent, potato starch; and quinoa, which can be used as a flour when baking cakes. Two other grains are usually tolerated by people with gluten-sensitive people, buckwheat and oat flour—sometimes used to add sweetness to baked goods.

Chapter 15 Summary

Some scientists believe that the tens of thousands of varieties of wheat are the primary major cause of obesity in the United States. By some accounts, a single slice of wheat bread has more dangerous sugars than several candy bars. The wheat grown today is deemed by some researchers as unnatural and unhealthful, vastly different from only a handful of natural varieties that were predominantly grown until the mid-1900s. Numerous medical professionals think the average American is unaware of this danger. Homeopaths believe that overweight people experience a much higher probability of getting cancer than thin individuals or people at their ideal weight. Lots of consumers claim that they have lost significant amounts of weight after refraining from wheat, even people who had previously exercised to no avail. More study is needed to determine if these negative claims regarding wheat are true. Meanwhile, this issue emerges as challenging for cancer patients because lots of doctors and dietitians tell them to eat lots of healthy fiber and especially wheat. Some of my patients and people on the Forsythe Anti-Cancer Diet might choose to avoid wheat for these reasons.

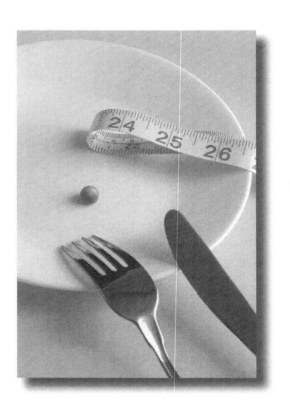

Chapter 16

Other
Culprits Identified

My research team has noticed that many of the top-selling, health-related electronic eBooks in recent years have also listed wheat as a major threat to public health. Most of these were published well before Davis' "Wheat Belly," which emerged as perhaps the most successful mainstream publication on the issue.

Sadly, in the meantime the top-selling eBooks on the secrets of "how to get a flat belly" have failed to get much recognition within the mainstream media. Perhaps the bulk of those publications want to generate significant profits, essentially while operating under the radar screen—to reduce the likelihood other publications will replicate this concept.

You see, while surfing the Internet, many consumers stumble across these "get-six-pack-abs" advertisements. At least from what we've reviewed, the bulk of those publications, which sell for as much as $49.95 a pop, reveal so-called insider information on the three primary foods that you should avoid in order to get a flat belly relatively fast.

Simply by avoiding these foods, the publications say, the vast majority of typical American consumers can quickly start to lose weight. This argument focuses squarely on the fact that the vast majority of consumers seem to eat foods bought quickly at the grocery store, paying little if any attention to what the meals contain.

Besides wheat, the other foods or meal additives that these publications say you should avoid are:

High-fructose Corn syrup: Blamed by some researchers as even more caloric or unhealthful than so-called refined sugars or white sugars, this substance is said to vastly boost weight in many people who incorrectly think that "I'm eating healthy."

Sweetened soy products: While a vast majority of us are told that soy is healthful and packed with essential proteins, this food reportedly contains far too many complex sugars for the body to efficiently process—ultimately resulting in excess weight.

Public Proclamations Abound

For the most part, these publications list the apparent proclamations of many people who say they quickly lost weight simply by simultaneously avoiding, wheat, high-fructose corn syrup and sweetened soy products.

To those of us whose primary objective is to prevent or control cancer, at least from what my researchers have seen, there is little if any mention of this disease in those reports or within for-profit publications.

Even so, as a physician I feel a responsibility to proclaim that if these recommendations hold any validity, simply avoiding those foods might very well play a potential role in preventing cancer. Once again, I cannot begin to stress enough the fact that big bellies serve as ovens or growth regions for the disease.

Meantime, I also caution my patients from jumping into every so-called "fad diet" that they see advertised or mentioned within the news media. From my view, the public's overall yearning for a sudden and effective weight loss miracle seems understandable. Sure enough, the U.S. Centers for Disease control and various health organizations keep warning the public that the overall obesity rate remains on a sharp upward trend.

Know What You Eat

Long before other physicians and health care professionals jumped onto this proverbial bandwagon, I became one of the earliest physicians to conclude that the jumps in cancer and weight gain occur largely because "we don't know what we're eating."

Compounding the problem, as stated earlier, many of the least expensive foods found in grocery stores contain additives suspected as harmful, highly fattening or potentially carcinogenic.

Struck by a steadily growing concern for this issue, during the summer of 2012, federal officials announced their prediction that during the next several decades up to half of all adults in many regions of the USA will be considered obese. Statisticians and health professionals believe that the biggest, most significant jumps in weight will occur in states considered as the poorest in America—particularly in Louisiana, Mississippi and other areas of the South.

Does this trend stem from the fact that low-income families buy as many of the cheapest, processed, wheat-laden foods that they can in order to survive? Just as disturbing, why weren't the dangers of potentially harmful food additive mentioned in any of these disturbing news articles?

National Security Becomes Threatened

Heightening my concerns and those of many other doctors, in the early fall of 2012 several retired U.S. military leaders including former generals and admirals joined to proclaim that obesity in America had become a "matter of national security."

According to widespread media reports, U.S. Defense Department officials had become gravely concerned that the obesity rate among young adults of recruitment age had soared to a whopping 25 percent.

If true, that means at least one out of every four potential military recruits was deemed too overweight to enter the military. Worsening matters, the officials feared, the overall rate of obesity among young recruits would continue jumping much higher.

Besides threatening the health of the overweight young adults, the trend decreased the ability of the U.S. government to quickly draft or recruit suitable, healthy young military personnel in the event of a sudden national emergency.

Healthy Meal Efforts Began Failing

Adding even more worries, during the same three-week period that officials announced the weight-gain trend and national security issues, high school, middle school and even some elementary school students nationwide began an informal, unorganized revolt.

Streams of media reports chronicled instances where frustrated children tossed much or all of their school-made lunches into the trash. The overall dissatisfaction among students emerged as school districts nationwide imposed new federally mandated healthy-meal regulations.

Under the guidance or at least recommendations of First Lady Michelle Obama, the meals contained more vegetables and fruits than before, at least according to some news accounts. Yet many children complained that the updated or reformatted menus were bland, tasteless and failed to leave them satisfied or "feeling full."

The seething conflict emerged as a serious dichotomy or

a blatant oxymoron at the very least. Had America's children become too addicted to sugars, sweets or potentially dangerous food additives? Or, did the federally mandated menus go too far, pushing us collectively to the point of becoming a "nanny state?"

As these flash-in-the-pan news reports gradually faded from the mainstream public consciousness, as a doctor, a husband, a father and a grandfather, I became increasingly concerned that the "overall national diet may have reached a point of insanity."

Bio-Engineered Foods Worsened the Problem

My professional concerns multiplied many-fold, during the same period when various behind-the-scenes, little-known news reports gave disturbing details of foods that had been "bio-engineered" without the public's knowledge—supposedly posing a grave potential threat to public health.

Everything came down to the fact that in various studies virtually 100 percent of laboratory rats that were fed only these bio-engineered foods developed cancer or tumors that were massive in size.

According to numerous research reports, all of this was done on the sly in order to increase the efficiency of massive food production via mega-corporations.

"To heck with the public—and full speed ahead," these greedy companies seemed to be saying to themselves. "Big bucks hail as our primary goal, and we're actually helping society by increasing the efficiency of the food-development industry."

Such mindless propaganda fails to satisfy those of us who became shocked upon learning that these corporations had started cramming the same crops that harmed laboratory rats into breakfast cereals. But why and how have these mega-corporations managed to get away with these greedy, extremely dangerous tactics while tampering with Mother Nature's natural plants?

Well, from my view on a national and international scale, the answer is simple: "Because they can, and no one including any federal agency is positioned to or willing to stop them. This trend is likely to continue unabated due primarily to the fact that—like Big Pharma—Big Food generates countless billions of dollars in annual revenues, made possible in part to the hogwash spewed by its hundreds or thousands of high-paid political lobbyists."

These professionals at double-speak pack the halls of the U.S. Congress in Washington, D.C., and within the catacombs of many governments worldwide, dead-set on ramming through their destructive agendas. While Big Food considers itself the winner in the financial sense, you as a consumer have become endangered far more than you might previously have realized—with cancer, diabetes and obesity emerging as your likely "war wounds."

Consumers Fight Back

Luckily, highly motivated consumers worldwide have started fighting back against Big Food's devilish strategies of developing and distributing dangerous genetically modified organisms— especially unnatural corn.

According to an article first printed at NaturalSociety.com, and later published at other Websites in the fall of 2012, consumer rights organizations in France and Russia were striving for legislation to ban the importation and use of genetically modified corn. Until that point, little of significance had been done within the United States to push for such legislation, perhaps due to Big Food's strong grip on our corrupt Congress.

Throughout 2011 and through the first half of 2012, consumers in California waged a heated battle to push for significant legislation. These political warriors publicly proclaimed their anger toward politicians, more concerned with getting re-elected than striving to protect public health. In what some behind-the-scene journalists described as the first effort of its kind, in November 2012 California voters had been expected to overwhelming pass a measure requiring that all labels on foods sold in the state specify if the products are genetically modified. Amazingly, however, the Proposition 37 initiative failed, possibly because voters were fooled by a $45 million anti-ballot campaign funded by Big Food. By comparison, consumers pushing for passage raised only $6.7 million to convince voters that the legislation made sense. Big Food companies like Monsanto had insisted such food labels would have been confusing to consumers. These firms argued that scientists have been unable to find significant evidence that genetically modified foods pose significant health risks. Even so, some health professionals had insisted such legislation would have been a major victory for consumers. Ultimately, from my perspective, huge conglomerate, multi-national corporations are likely to win such political fights in the future because average consumers have much less financial resources to saturate the media with effective advertising.

The Golden state often leads the way in such legislation, with a population and industry rivaling most nations. Prior to defeat, some consumer rights organizations expressed their hope that passage of the labeling requirement in California would motivate other states and Congress to approve similar legislation.

The Legislative Fight Erupted

Adding a proverbial cherry to the top of their proverbial celebration cake, in France the opponents of Big Food's genetic-modification systems pushed for a worldwide ban on such crops pending the outcome of further study on the issue. Ultimately, these consumers say, an initial study in France found a "serious link between the consumption" of a mega-food corporation's genetically modified crops and big tumors. The genetic modification process enables the crops to withstand the ravages of highly dangerous, chemical-laden weed-killing sprays.

If foods containing genetically modified organisms are properly labeled, "the simple fact of the matter is that less people will buy them," the NaturalSociety.com article said. "As of right now, very few people are even aware of what they are putting in their mouth. In fact, if the public knew that they were consuming GMOs (genetically modified organisms) that are linked to massive tumors and organ failure, the overwhelming majority would abandon such products. Without labeling, however, they have no idea."

The California initiative's campaign manager Gary Raskin told the publication that huge corporations like "Monsanto, DuPont and Coca-Cola do not want Californians to know what's really in their food and drinks, because they fear consumers will turn away from their (the companies') genetically engineered ingredients and pesticides that go with them."

In addition, the publication says, the vast majority of consumers are unaware when they're eating highly poisonous mercury contained in certain genetically modified foods, or artificial sweeteners associated with at least 42 diseases.

When and if such required labeling starts, the report said, "then change would occur—change that includes forcing manufacturers to abandon these ingredients in order to stay profitable. And, after all, Monsanto's number-one goal is profit. This is a company that has been caught running 'slave-like' working conditions in which 'employees' were forced to buy only from the company store, and were not allowed to leave the area, or their pay would be withheld."

Beware of Food Labels

Long before the widespread push for such mandatory labeling legislation, for several decades I have warned my patients to be wary of the apparent accuracy of such mandatory notices.

Under the guidance and stipulations of the U.S. Federal Food and Drug Administration, commonly called the "FDA," the makers and distributors of vitamin supplements and food packaging are required to list the so-called percentages each pill or serving has of the agency's "recommended daily allowance" for vitamins and minerals.

But many homeopaths and even some mainstream physicians universally agree that such so-called good or minimum-nutrition levels are artificially set at incorrect levels. Thus, a person might need far more or even less than packaging or labels might indicate.

As if this weren't already enough to intensify concerns, required labels on foods fail to come anywhere close to telling the complete story. For instance, perhaps because the U.S. government is "in bed with" huge corporations, some labels shockingly are allowed to list "zero trans fats," when in fact a food might contain less than 0.5 grams of such unhealthful substances per serving.

Worsening matters to potentially critical levels, the amounts that food producers consider as a single "serving" might invariably become far less than a typical person would eat. Thus, unsuspecting consumers sometimes ultimately get far less of the vitamins and minerals that they actually need, while also ingesting far more potentially harmful substances without knowing they're eating such dangerous foods.

How Many Vitamins and Minerals are Recommended?

Most people know that the government recommends a "required daily allowance" or RDA of specific vitamins and minerals. By law, through a required packaging and labeling process, distributors of foods, vitamins and minerals must specify the percentage of these substances that a particular product contains.

However, in all these instances—everything from cereal boxes to milk cartons—the term "100 percent" refers to the *least* amount of a vitamin or mineral that physicians deem necessary to sustain good health. Medical professionals consider these minimum levels as the lowest amount essential to prevent a wide variety of diseases including scurvy, rickets, pellagra, beriberi, pernicious anemia and many other affiliations.

When developing these FDA requirements, medical professionals used nutritional studies that were conducted as far back as the 1940s. However, at the time scientists and physicians lacked precise methods of testing and determining levels of vitamins and minerals in tissue and blood. Modern equipment gives much more accurate results.

Sadly, the minimum RDA levels specified by the government fail to meet the human body's requirements, especially amid the increased onslaught of serious cancer, severe cardiovascular disease, environmental toxins and virulent viruses or bacterial illnesses. Severe stress that people suffer in today's society compounds these problems.

The RDA and optimal daily allowances can vary significantly for specific vitamins and minerals. For instance, the RDA for Vitamin C is 60 milligrams per day, compared to an optimal daily allowance of about 1,000 milligrams daily for the same substance. Vitamins A and E are among many individual vitamins and minerals with optimal daily doses significantly higher than the RDA listed for each of them.

Chapter 16 Summary

Besides wheat, numerous online eBooks selling for up to $49.95 each also list high-fructose corn syrup and sweetened soy products as foods to avoid in order to lose weight. Some people insist they've lost many pounds with this strategy. Sadly, many of these items are in food labels, so many consumers are unaware they're eating them. More research is needed. Many of these meals are sold relatively cheaply in low-income regions where obesity is increasing. Consumers have fought back, making some strides in requiring better food labeling and some prohibitions of harmful food additives—but much more still needs to be done on the political front. All along, food labels are often inaccurate, and the federal government's recommendations on how much specific vitamins people should eat daily are often vague or inaccurate.

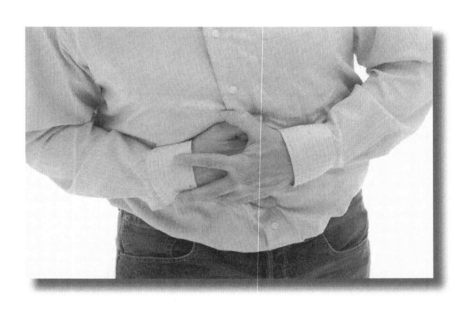

Chapter 17

Respect and Help Your Intestines

Now that you know the potentially risky health risks—including the possibility of cancer—imposed by Big Food and Big Pharma, you should take decisive action to take control of your cancer or to prevent such a disease.

So, for my patients or to anyone wanting to minimize cancer risks, I strongly urge taking a proactive approach to minimizing the effects of toxins on the body.

The overall sense of urgency in this initial task becomes even clearer when taking into account that various factors other than Big Food processes can substantially increase your potential toxic load. Disturbingly, many of us lack adequate amounts of healthy bacteria. This danger sometimes intensifies when drinking chlorinated water. As if all this weren't already enough to cause concern, the excessive or even infrequent use of antibiotics sometimes robs the body of microorganisms that help ward off or fight diseases including cancer.

An improperly functioning intestinal tract can prevent the body from absorbing adequate or necessary nutrients.

I've discovered instances among many patients where the intestinal wall becomes so porous due to improper nutrition or symptoms of various diseases that certain large proteins shoot right through the gut and straight into the blood stream.

These problems, in turn, can lead to extreme difficulties with inflammation or even allergies, generating hurdles to overcome in regaining good health or in battling cancer. Such intestinal "leakage" problems occasionally are triggered by everything from toxins, drugs, and stress to infections.

Healthy Intestines Serve as a Key

Fully cognizant of these risk factors or challenges, you and your physician should always pay close attention to the function of the intestines—particularly when treating cancer. This task can become formidable for patients who have undergone extensive chemotherapy, losing their physical strength and in some cases wrecking the digestive tract's ability to function at peak efficiency.

While always aware of these potentially critical factors, the best doctors, nurses and patients realize that both the small and large intestines play a far more important role than just the transporting of waste products from the body.

As a highly complex organism, the lower digestive tract also serves a vital role in your body's ability to absorb nutrients, while helping and strengthening the immune system. Without these important functions working at peak efficiency, for the most part a cancer patient cannot fully regain optimal good health. Adding to the complexity, I believe that patients who have not suffered from cancer experience a greater propensity to eventually get this disease in a variety of forms if the digestive tract malfunctions.

"The success or failure of your intestines dictates the quality of your overall health," I tell patients. "In fact, without the proper functioning of these organs various bodily functions can stop operating right—everything from the brain to the formulation of certain necessary naturally, internally produced hormones."

Respect Warning Signs

All cancer patients and even healthy individuals need to watch for a wide variety of warning signs that might indicate their intestines lack adequate functions.

The wide variety of potential signals range from a slow memory to immunity problems, diarrhea or even stools that contain undigested particles of food. The vast range of other potential problems spans everything from iron deficiency to arthritis symptoms, constipation, asthma or a vast array of skin conditions such as rosacea, eczema, acne and psoriasis.

When such conditions occur I often order a stool panel analysis to determine the gut's function levels. Potential results might span everything from pathogens harming the small intestines to yeast outgrowths, or even discoveries of cancer within the intestines or other organs. Some results reveal that the body has inadequate amounts of stomach acid, which—contrary to the mistaken belief of many people—is not the primary cause of heartburn. To the contrary, the usual cause of heartburn is the exact opposite, an insufficient amount of stomach acids.

Observe Your Stools

Although always cautioning patients never to serve as their own physicians striving to reach a self-diagnosis, they're encouraged to observe the quality of their own stools. Although not scientific in nature, such amateur checks can help determine:

Poor digestion: Large, heavy or misshapen stools that sink to the bottom of the bowl almost as if heavy anchors, lots of spattering in small spots scattered around the toilet, or the necessity to push hard due to constipation—which sometimes occurs sporadically.

Good digestion: The stool is long and curled like a snake or a huge but soft banana, lightly floating atop the bowl like a floatation device or a balloon floating on air. The "going" process is smooth, easy and effortless.

When the digestive process seems to be working well, the so-called "good" signals might indicate that the person is eating a proper, well-balanced diet that enables the body to easily handle its digestion chores. Just as important, these same positive signs also can show that the individual's digestive system is—or at least seems to be—in relatively good health.

Conversely, the "bad" indicators might signify that a person has either recently eaten inadvisable or unhealthy foods such as processed meals, or that perhaps the individual might be suffering from some sort of underlying malfunction within the digestive systems. Only a trained medical professional can reach such conclusions.

Links Between Cancers and Food

All these factors can help point to the initial discovery of cancer or to the development of physical challenges while treating the disease.

Meantime, of course, the issue of what foods to eat and to avoid for the particular patient's needs also arises. But before delving into what general food types you'll need in order to improve the intestines' ability to handle toxic burdens, you must understand the basic criteria for either maintaining or regaining healthy digestion.

Every step of the way through your recovery from cancer,

your attempts to beat the disease or to prevent its recurrence, your goal should be to enable the body to easily digest what you eat, fully absorb proper nutrients, and ultimately to "assimilate" all these various substances that the body needs to thrive at optimal levels. When performed right, eating as recommended, you'll give your body a "fighting chance" to effectively battle or prevent cancer, without having to deal with excessive levels of toxins.

Whether in the recovery or prevention mode, your goal should be to keep foods moving steadily through the body, all while effortlessly removing waste. All this should be done without suffering digestive ailments.

For many, adequate amounts of fibers serve as the key to efficiently moving food, nutrients and waste through the body. Everything from apples to bananas and certain grains can help the body perform these chores with ease.

When and if this naturally occurring "enter and exit" process seems to stall, rather than relying on laxative medications I'm among physicians who recommend foods that contain naturally occurring amounts of magnesium. Common and easily obtainable magnesium sources can include everything from bananas, dark-green, leafy vegetables, nuts, pumpkin seeds, whole grains and blackstrap molasses.

Consumers and patients should remain aware that medications can curtail, prevent or counteract the potential laxative benefits of foods high in magnesium. Partly for these reasons, some doctors recommend, administer or prescribe supplements high in easily absorbed magnesium.

Respect Belly Bugs

Did you know that in healthy people the stomach and particularly the small and large intestines contain up to four pounds of bacteria?

Like this or not, when healthy your body contains literally hundreds of trillions of bacteria within the intestines. So, in order to maintain or regain good health the Forsythe Anti-Cancer Diet concentrates on foods deemed ideal for enabling these healthy bacteria to work at peak efficiency.

Any failure to achieve this essential goal could slow down or stall a cancer patient's overall recovery. You see, at least by some accounts the healthy bacteria within your intestines number far more than the entire amount of cells within your body.

"You have powerful and necessary, naturally occurring allies within your body," I tell some cancer patients. "Without their valuable assistance, your probability for a full recovery might become minimized."

Understandably, lots of people who previously were unfamiliar with these basics of human biology become fascinated. These patients sometimes perk up, highly inquisitive upon learning that the intestinal tracts of healthy people contain upwards of 400 or more organisms deemed "beneficial and necessary" to good health.

Lined throughout the intestinal tract, these organisms help the body's digestion process. Just as important, these bacteria also play a critical role in producing a wide variety of enzymes that your body needs to survive.

As if all this weren't already enough to impress patients, these critical organisms also enable the body to produce B vitamins that help the liver's detoxification process. Intestinal bacteria also produce Vitamin K, necessary for the body to modify proteins essential for bones and other tissues.

Rescue and Help These Essential Bacteria

Especially for cancer patients who have become seriously ill, as an integrative medical oncologist I become highly motivated to prescribe or recommend foods or supplements beneficial to "good" intestinal bacteria.

For many thousands of years, doctors and even countless families from many societies have realized the power of certain fermented foods to strengthen or assist these vital biological substances. Loaded with healthful bacteria, the ideal foods within this category include certain yogurts, plus other foods that have fermented in the production or preparation process such as sauerkraut or Kimchi first prevalent in East Asia.

Yet within modern society farm animals intended for eventual use as human food are fed relatively new substances or medicines such as hormones and prescription antibiotics. When eating meat, people eventually get contaminated with these potentially cancerous substances.

Intensifying this potential for imbalance, some unhealthful organisms also occasionally thrive within the intestines. When an imbalance called "dysbiosis" strikes, various negative symptoms can adversely impact numerous areas of the body such as the eyes, vagina, nose, mouth and ears.

Needless to say, any effort to optimize the performance of intestinal bacteria could possibly become particularly challenging due to these potential hurdles. For obvious reasons, some scientists and doctors call these potentially harmful bacteria "opportunistic organisms." These problems sometimes generate "hostile bacteria," or opportunistic yeast that actively and aggressively strives to consume as many sugars as possible—usually yearning for carbohydrates. Patients with too much of these unhealthful yeasts within their intestines sometimes crave excessive amounts of high-calorie carbohydrates like pizza, bread, crackers and pasta.

This domino effect in turn often results in excessive weight gain, generating big bellies that greatly increase the person's probability of eventually getting cancer. This situation becomes exacerbated for patients who already have the disease, while the unhealthful yeast continues making them crave the foods that made them obese.

Probiotics Enter the Scene

With increasing frequency people worldwide use probiotics to load their intestines with beneficial bacteria, in hopes of counteracting or eliminating the effects of "bad" organisms. Helpful probiotics usually come in the form of fermented foods like yogurt and sauerkraut. In many instances a cancer patient's "gut problems" sparked by unhelpful bacteria becomes so intense that eating sufficient amounts of probiotics becomes challenging. Similar hurdles often emerge among people without cancer as well, conditions ignited by a variety of ailments.

When this happens, my clinic often refers or provides patients with probiotic supplements taken multiple times daily. Similar strategies often become part of the game plan even before symptoms of potential hostile bacteria become severe, particularly amid intense treatments for cancer.

This way the patient's "good bacteria" gets protected, increasing the probability that medications will have minimal effect on the body's ability to absorb vital nutrients.

Every step through cancer treatment, as an integrative medical oncologist, my primary objectives include enabling the patient to maintain as much energy and vigor as possible. That's why on occasion I also consider employing "saccharomyces boulardii," yeast that French scientist Henri Boulard isolated from various fruits in 1923. Homeopaths agree that this ingredient often hailed as the "yeast of yeasts" can maintain a significant role as a probiotic in enabling the small and large intestines to strengthen, to rejuvenate and to maintain healthful levels of natural flora.

Although this essential yeast is hailed as a healthful natural substance, you should only use it under the continual monitoring and direction of a health professional or dietician. According to some researchers, this unique yeast can generate problems for people whose immune systems are suppressed. Besides localized infections, other potential problems include systematic blood infections or "fungemia," when fungi or yeasts enter the blood. Only a certified health professional can diagnose and treat these ailments, particularly fungemia, which sometimes strikes oncology patients or even people who are using intravenous catheters or those suffering from neutropenia, an abnormally low level of white blood cells—necessary in fighting infections and diseases including cancer.

These are among a handful of many reasons why a single, one-diet-fits-all system never works universally for every cancer patient. Even so, as your own individualized anti-cancer diet is developed and implemented, always remember that an appropriate probiotic regimen can emerge as an essential tool in increasing the likelihood of gaining or regenerating good health.

Understand Basics of Probiotics

The World Health Organization considers probiotics so important that its medical professionals insist that such organisms are essential to good health. Even more important, from my perspective, such bacteria also often become doubly important for the treatment of cancer patients.

Homeopaths and dieticians appreciate the fact that microbes considered as probiotics are often in the form of bifidobacteria and lactic acid bacteria. Bifidobacteria is frequently found within the mouths, vaginas and gastrointestinal tracts of mammals. While this might seem strange to the lay person, the food industry considers this segment of bacteria as an important probiotic for generating beneficial health.

For cancer patients, lactic acid bacteria can emerge as a formidable weapon in helping the intestines and ultimately overall digestion. As a homeopath and an oncologist, I appreciate the fact that lactic acid bacteria are "acid-tolerant."

This attribute grows in significance because generally cancers thrive in acidic environments. On a molecular level, the primary attributes of lactic acid bacteria are often generated by the decomposition process of certain plants.

Often called "LAB" by scientists, these amazing bacteria can out-compete other organisms, essential within the food industry.

According to a 2001 article in the "American Journal of Clinical Nutrition," some strains of LAB are effective in preventing or inhibiting the formation of cancers that can occur when ingesting red meat. A February 2000 "Journal of Nutrition" article said researchers found evidence that LAB acted against the colon cancers of rodents, although this bacteria's impact on similar disease within humans remained inconclusive. Just as promising, according to various published reports LAB might have anti-carcinogenic attributes by reducing certain enzyme activity. In fact, according to a separate article in the same 2000 "Journal of Nutrition" issue, in one study researchers observing a specific population of people detected lower instances of colon cancer among consumers who ate fermented dairy products.

Researchers were unable to find specific evidence that such foods universally prevent colon cancer. More extensive research should be done on this issue while doctors, dietitians and patients consider adding fermented dairy products to at least some of their food recommendations.

Appreciate Potential Health Benefits

The many health benefits of probiotic foods and supplements also lure people suffering from a variety of ailments other than cancer. Researchers in a wide variety of studies have found at least moderate or even substantial benefits from probiotics, helping people who suffer from many ailments, ranging from high blood pressure and cholesterol problems to immunity challenges.

For oncology issues, I'm particularly interested in the ability of probiotic foods to energize and rekindle the body's immune systems.

Protections against disease and potentially deadly infections like pneumonia become critical, particularly if a cancer patient loses strength or immune functions falter during or immediately after chemotherapy.

Some researchers believe they may have found evidence that probiotics strengthen and fortify the body's natural immune functions. This becomes critically important when probiotics accelerate the body's natural production of essential T-cells, necessary fighters in battling bodily invaders like cancer, according to various research reports including a 2003 article in "Clinical Microbiology."

A 2010 "Science Daily" report goes even further, stating that probiotics might help patients maintain the ability to fight disease, protecting their immune systems.

Protect Your Intestinal Lining

While remaining appreciative of the many benefits of probiotics, all patients with serious health issues—particularly people with cancer—need to eat foods deemed ideal in preventing the intestinal tract from leaking. When at peak levels, the intestinal tract's lining performs two essential chores required for good health:

Pass: Allow foods that have been efficiently processed or digested elsewhere in the body to easily move through the body to the bowel movement phase.

Block: Prohibit dangerous substances from entering the intestines, such as pathogens or infectious agents that contain harmful virus, fungus and bacteria that could lead to a variety of diseases including cancer. The intestines of healthy people block substances that the body's pathological mechanisms deem as too large to generate any benefit.

A potentially hazardous health condition that doctors call "leaky gut" occasionally develops due to excessive toxins, or resulting from the ingestion of medicines that generate more stress than the body can naturally handle.

For patients with "leaky guts" the dangers can become formidable, especially when the intestines lose their natural abilities to block dangerous substances. Worsening matters, this condition can cause the overall immune system to go haywire.

Potential complications sometimes include autoimmune problems, symptoms that mirror or reflect actual allergies, or even inflammation that can cause excess pain to cancer patients while also hampering their recoveries.

To combat a leaky gut, under the direction of a health care professional or herbalist who works in association with your doctor, you should consider taking healthful herbs like slippery elm, yarrow, chamomile, kudzu, and marshmallow roots. These can play essential roles in healing or reformulating essential bacteria.

Just as important, cancer patients with leaky guts should strive to avoid toxic foods, while also eating adequate amounts of "prebiotics," usually fibers eaten by healthy bacteria within the intestines. Along with plenty of vegetables and fruit, these tactics are needed to enable the intestines to accept or block the appropriate substances.

Patients who drink alcohol open the doorway to continued problems, hampering the digestive system and wrecking the body's ability to block and remove toxins. Additional roadblocks can emerge when using unnecessary antibiotics, drinking chlorinated, unfiltered water, or using drugs that ravage the gut lining.

Understand "Leaky Gut" Issues

On a molecular level, a "leaky gut" occurs when "tight junctions" or TJs become barriers between the digestive tract's intestinal epithelial walls.

At least according to various published reports and research papers, scientists blame "leaky gut" for sometimes sparking numerous other health problems besides those already mentioned. While these research efforts might individually and collectively seem inconclusive to some physicians, the listed potential diseases include Type 1 diabetes, asthma, allergies, and autism. Unproven theories also suggest adverse effects on patients who suffer heart failure.

Specifically, as an oncologist I'm concerned with the potential for a "leaky gut" to hinder cancer treatments, causing unnecessary or unforeseen complications.

Rather than using unnatural anti-oxidative or anti-inflammatory drugs produced by pharmaceutical companies, some Homeopaths consider natural substances often deemed effective for these conditions. Among the nutrients or food properties mentioned often here:

Glutamine: Frequent or common natural dietary sources include parsley, beans, spinach, milk, beef, fish, chicken beets, wheat, cabbage and dairy products.

157

Zinc: This metallic element is available in certain supplements or most over-the-counter vitamins. Among its many potential benefits, according to some researchers, is an "anti-oxidant" attribute—preventing the oxidation reactions that ultimately can lead to "free radicals," an internal biological process that often leads to the formation of cancers. According to a wide variety of published reports, foods that contain the highest concentrations of zinc include veal liver, oysters, toasted wheat germ, roasted pumpkin and squash seeds, low-fat roast beef, dark chocolate or chocolate powders, lamb, dried watermelon seeds, crab and peanuts.

Acetylcysteine: Usually obtained as nutritional supplements or pharmaceutical drugs, it's sometimes used in cough medicines thanks to its ability to loosen bonds within and to liquefy mucus. Some companies selling acetylcystine within supplements claim that this mucolytic agent performs antioxidant functions while protecting the liver. Besides yogurt, common dietary sources of acetyclcystine are derived from animal products like cottage cheese, pork, ricotta, chicken, milk, turkey, and eggs. Frequently mentioned plant sources reportedly include lentils, red peppers, wheat germ, garlic, granola, Brussels sprouts, broccoli and onions.

Chapter 17 Summary

Avoiding and recovering from cancer hinges on the vibrant health of the intestines. People can observe the quality of their stools for warning signs of possible intestinal problems. Unhealthy intestines are sometimes unable to handle the toxic overloads generated by unhealthy foods. The intestines are loaded with several pounds of bacteria. The "good" intestinal bacteria helps in the digestive process, enabling the body to process and eliminate potential carcinogens. "Bad" bacteria creates a biological environment that enables carcinogens to thrive. Probiotic foods can help good bacteria thrive and strengthen the intestines, while destroying unhealthy bacteria. Probiotics fortify the body's natural processes of allowing foods that have been efficiently processed and digested to exit the body via bowel movements. Effective probiotics also help the body block dangerous substances from entering the intestines, a defect sometimes called "leaky gut." Foods often deemed helpful in addressing "leaky guts" include slippery elm, yarrow, marshmallow roots, chamomile and kudzu. Homeopaths can recommend specific probiotic foods to strengthen helpful bacteria.

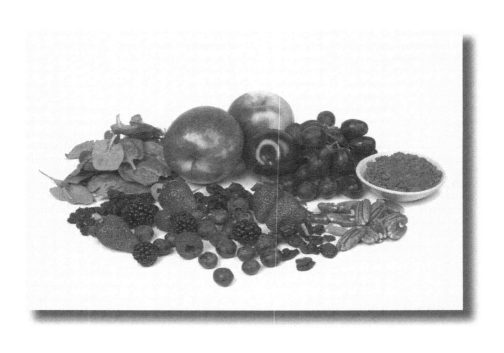

Chapter 18

Eat
Antioxidant Foods

Eat a variety of foods deemed to have antioxidant attributes. These qualities enable the body to fight or to remove free radicals, which on a molecular level are unpaired ions, molecules or atoms.

When left unabated or unchecked in excess quantities, free radicals often cause injury or death to numerous cells while generating a propensity for the formation of cancer. According to some researchers, the danger becomes so serious that just a single free-radical atom can eventually lead to full-blown, malignant stage IV cancer. Other potential health problems reputedly ignited on occasion by free radicals include some instances of stroke, myocardial infractions, and diabetes.

On a molecular level, researchers strongly believe that free radicals generate mutations by first damaging the body's DNA or genetic instructions that map out a person's entire biological structure. The mutations form when certain elements or segments of the body's cell structure inadvertently change the person's individualized, natural DNA genomic sequence.

This problem then hampers or breaks the body's normally efficient "cell cycle," a continuous lifelong process where cells divide—usually a healthy, and necessary system in which cells naturally and predictably create mirror versions of themselves. Within healthy people, when the cell cycle works efficiently throughout the entire body, an individual is often capable of living for several decades or even more than a century.

Well, everything goes off kilter when free radicals hidden within a person's cellular structure create unwanted mutations that generate cancer. Instead of creating mirror images of themselves when dividing, cells form irregular mutations that become cancer. Steadily over time in some individuals the situation worsens as cancer reaches full-blown stages, sometimes metastasizing to various organs.

What Causes Free Radicals?

The initial onset of free radicals within an individual has been blamed on everything from cooking meats on grills at fast food restaurants to unnatural food additives and radiation from cell phones. Faced with worries that they're getting blamed for creating food-based and drug-induced free radicals, Big Food and Big Pharma are fighting back within the political realm and in the media war in hopes of convincing us that they are not to blame.

Nonetheless, thanks largely to consumer advocacy groups and civil court actions, various substances, chemicals and specially prepared foods have been either officially or unofficially labeled as "carcinogens." Generally, these are foods, objects or molecular reactions deemed likely to sharply increase your risk of getting cancer by entering the body's cells, where DNA gets damaged.

When left untreated or undetected, mutations resulting from damaged DNA can lead to cancers that generate what scientists give the chilling label "programmed cell death."

Sometimes referred to by the acronym PCD, this process

normally occurs as a pre-planned, predictable and even a necessary ongoing process in many organisms—even within healthy humans. Within healthy people, cells naturally die as they're efficiently replaced by new versions of the same structures. But the process gets off kilter when mutations spawned from free radicals damage DNA so severely that the problem becomes difficult to repair.

Some Carcinogens Occur Naturally

At least according to some published reports, carcinogens occasionally occur naturally or due to the inappropriate, ill-advised methods in storing certain foods including peanut butter, nuts and grains. By no means is this statement meant as an indication that you should avoid such foods, which many physicians generally considered healthful when stored properly.

Even so, a microbial carcinogen that occurs naturally when stored with grains, generated by the fungus Aspergillus flavus—a relatively common mold—is aflotoxin. This reigns as an extremely serious material in the mycotoxin class, a notoriously toxic carcinogenic chemical derived from fungi.

For these reasons people without cancer and those with the disease should strive to buy grains, breads and nuts only from reputable food producers. Amateur farmers new to the agricultural industry or who lack adequate training can inadvertently cause the growth of or the spread of carcinogenic foods.

All along, consumers also need to remain aware that as members of the Aspergillus class, aflatoxins are widespread and even common throughout nature.

Adding to the dangers, aflatoxins can actually contaminate grains during pre-harvest periods, long before the storage process.

Far more catastrophic than a corny plot in a B-grade 1950s horror movie, farm animals sometimes eat contaminated grains.

These same animals, possibly including dairy cows, eventually pass these carcinogens further through the food chain via their milk. Shockingly, according to numerous reports, various tests on a variety of products and foods ranging from cooking oil, olive oil and peanut butter show that from 48 percent to 80 percent of those foods contained levels of aflatoxin that exceed what the FDA considers safe.

Dangers Increase Concern

Patients developing, starting or continuing a Forsythe Anti-Cancer Diet regimen also need to know that countless other verified or suspected carcinogens exist. Once patients understand the basics of these widespread, formidable dangers, they quickly get a better understanding of why and how certain foods are needed for their specific needs.

Just some of the many other carcinogens include:

Asbestos: Officially listed by many governments and health organizations as carcinogenic, this naturally occurring substance was formerly used commercially on a widespread basis—often in home and commercial building construction. The most serious diseases caused by inhalation of asbestos fibers include the malignant lung cancer mesothelioma.

EDB: This naturally occurring organic compound often found in the ocean, with the scientific name ethylene dibromide, is created by kelp and algae. Once used frequently as a pesticide, this carcinogen has been suspected of causing birth defects.

Dioxins: Along with highly toxic dioxin-like compounds, these substances deemed as persistent organic pollutants and environmental pollutants have been created for industrial use. Scientists blame dioxins for generating tumors and damaging the body's important glandular systems that regulate hormones and bloodstream function.

Benzene: A natural organic chemical compound and
a "petrochemical" from crude oil, this colorless and highly
flammable liquid is an important ingredient in gasoline. Besides
forming cancer, it's often blamed for bone marrow failure and
other diseases.

Kepone: Involved as a controversial, notorious and banned
insecticide, now prohibited throughout the western world, this
colorless, solid organochlorine compound was produced in such
massive quantities that people and wildlife in widespread regions
were exposed. Prostate cancer is among the most prevalent
diseases caused by kepone.

The Need for Antioxidant Diets Intensifies
The widespread and pervasive need for all-out use of the
Forsythe Anti-Cancer Diet becomes even more urgent when
acknowledging that even more carcinogens are continually
threatening your health.

Everything from industrial smoke to cigarettes and second-
hand smoke breathed in public places sharply increases your
probability of getting cancer.

One of the most disturbing dangers that many people seem
unaware of involves formaldehyde used for embalming and the
production of plastics. In fact, the third most widely used plastic,
polyvinyl chloride—commonly called PVC, is often used within
everyday materials like clothing and upholstery.

It's also used in home construction for everything from
pipes to electric cables, window frames and sills, and plumbing.
Although plastics are generally considered durable, over time
micro-particles called "micro-plastics" by scientists can reach
surfaces and the air—seriously endangering people.

While danger levels remain in dispute, many consumers have urged bans on PVC within plastics of shower curtains and car interiors. Several Japanese car companies stopped using PVC plastics in 2007.

Dangers of Food Preparation

Some research has shown that up to 35 percent of all cancer in humans is generated by improperly prepared foods, according to a 1981 report in the "Journal of the National Cancer Institute."

Consumers need to know that improperly preparing or cooking certain foods can create carcinogens. According to a 1999 article in the "Journal of the National Cancer Institute," the grilling or barbecuing of meats sometimes forms miniscule amounts of potent carcinogens. The report says smoking cigarettes is equally dangerous.

Scientists concluded that such cooking methods generate a propensity for the body to transform certain enzymes into epoxide, which subsequently and permanently becomes attached to DNA. This, in turn, generates tumors that can evolve into full-blown cancer.

According to a 2004 report by the National Cancer Institute, heating meats in a microwave for two minutes to three minutes prior to the grilling process can remove certain precursors from this food—decreasing the possibility that carcinogens will be created on the grill.

Various news reports and published articles in the early 1990s told of National Cancer Institute studies showing that people eating rare or medium-rare meats had a lower instance of stomach cancer than individuals whose meats were cooked well or medium-well.

Adding to the complexity of this issue, many processed foods and pre-cooked foods contain a carcinogenic, nitrosamine—

which scientists have known since 1956 as a cause of liver tumors in rats. According to a 2006 report in the "World Journal of Gastroenterology," a study indicated that nitrosamine increases the risk of stomach cancer. Unless effective treatments or surgery is employed in a timely manner, stomach cancer often becomes deadly because symptoms usually do not become evident until advanced stages of the disease.

Additional controversy arises when considering Food Standards Agency reports that indicate a carcinogen gets created during the overheating or frying of foods like potato chips and French fries. Media reports indicate studies on this issue are ongoing.

As if these factors weren't already enough to spark concern, smoking meat and fish also increases the potential development of carcinogenic hydrocarbons.

In addition, significant concentrations of another possible carcinogen, acrylamide, can get generated when broiling, grilling or baking foods when high starch levels form a toasty crust, according to a 2002 agricultural food chemistry journal. Consumers need to realize that acylamide is a highly toxic chemical compound used in numerous industrial processes as a water-soluble thickener, integral in various uses including papermaking, producing permanent press fabrics, wastewater treatment and the production of dyes.

Largely because scientists have known that median doses of acylamide are lethal to rabbits, controversy erupted in 2002 when consumers learned that the compound is sometimes used in the cooking of starchy foods. Studies reported in "Nature" and "Chemistry World" showed that the natural amino acid asparagine and the reducing of sugars like glucose and fructose may produce acrylamide while baking or frying.

Separate, unaffiliated and independent reports by a variety of agencies and researchers in recent decades detail the discoveries of acrylamide in wide varieties of foods that are generally considered healthy. These include whole wheat bread, roasted almonds, cocoa powder, coffee, black olives, dried pairs, prunes, and prune juice.

Meantime, numerous reports generated by a variety of separate studies seemed to indicate little or no cancer symptoms among people who ate foods containing acrylamide.

Even so, a 2007 report by the University of California at Berkeley concluded that high doses of this substance given orally to rats caused tumors. A European study on food toxicants from 2003 to 2007 concluded that acrylamide poses an enhanced risk to humans.

Determined to enable the public to learn of risks posed by acrylamide, in 2005 William Westwood "Bill" Lockyear—then California's attorney general—filed a lawsuit targeting the state's biggest makers of potato chips and French fries. In a 2008 settlement the industry agreed to cut in half the amount of this chemical compound in the foods. However, huge corporations still use acrylamide to produce herbicides on an industrial scale.

Additional Dangers from Cooking

Especially when cooking at home during an anti-cancer food regimen, you also should always remain cognizant that by not cooking dairy products you might sharply increase the natural anti-cancer attributes of such foods.

For instance, the risk of colorectal cancer gets reduced after eating un-pasteurized, uncooked dairy products, at least according to research at the University of Toronto.

However, such findings fail to convince the U.S. Food and Drug Administration, which never found scientific evidence that raw milk enhances the body's risk of disease.

The pros and cons erupting from diverse studies on the possible dangers imposed by certain cooking methods reached another boiling point when a 1997 report in a national scientific publication showed that glycotoxins can be produced when heating fats or proteins with sugars.

Benefit from Anti-carcinogens

The overall Forsythe Anti-Cancer strategy focuses on the wide spectrum of verified and suspected carcinogens. A primary weapon here entails all foods or helpful chemicals deemed as having "anti-carcinogen" attributes.

In terms that lay people can easily understand, an anti-carcinogen is anything that reduces or eliminates the possibility of cancer. Just as important, especially from the perspective of people who have the disease, some anti-carcinogens also have been shown by various studies to reduce this condition's severity.

On a scientific level, patients striving to prevent or to effectively manage their cancers should ingest foods or supplements that clinical studies indicate have a strong propensity of enabling them to achieve these vital health-oriented goals.

Even before launching any necessary or recommended changes in their eating habits, people striving to minimize their chances of getting cancer should avoid foods that are listed or suspected carcinogens—or that contain substances posing such dangers. Steering clear of these substances becomes doubly important for those already having cancer.

Concentrate on Flavonoids and Vitamins

To make sure your overall diet is anti-carcinogenic, you'll need to develop a diet regimen loaded with vitamins and flavonoids. Specified minerals or extremely minute amounts of recommended minerals also play essential roles, particularly those listed in the anti-cancer realm such as zinc and selenium.

Luckily for people with cancer, flavonoids are found abundantly throughout nature and as crops. These anti-carcinogenic foods generally are easy for the body to digest and to absorb in large amounts, thanks largely to their extremely low toxicity. This is in contrast to foods within the opposite spectrum, alkaloids such as poppy that contains morphine, the primary ingredient in heroin and extremely dangerous painkillers.

Literally dozens or perhaps hundreds of scientific studies indicate that flavonoid plants are likely to modify or offset the potential effects of carcinogens. From my perspective as a homeopath and as a physician, this makes flavonoids ideal and powerful players for any effective, well-rounded anti-carcinogen food regimen.

Added benefits from flavonoids can sometimes address adverse symptoms of either cancer or various treatments for the disease. Besides its strength in correcting or preventing diarrhea, flavonoid plants can help battle inflammation that often afflicts cancer patients—while also addressing or counteracting allergies.

Additional blessings from flavonoids emerge, according to some studies, thanks to their strength at inhibiting DNA mutations that would otherwise ultimately generate solid tumors or leukemia.

Foods Loaded with Flavonoid

The foods packed with healthy amounts of flavonoid—sometimes called "bioflavonoid"—are abundant and varied, enabling those employing Forsythe Anti-Cancer Diet strategies to enjoy a wide variety of meals and snacks.

One of the most popular foods here is low-sugar or non-white sugar dark chocolate that has a cocoa content of at least 70 percent.

Rounding out the mix are onions, especially the red variety.

Other popular and abundant high-flavonoid foods include berries, white tea and green tea, sea-buckthorn (found abundantly in Asia and Europe), red wine, parsley, pulses and ginkgo biloba.

Many citrus fruits are packed full of these vital anti-carcinogen attributes. Besides their strength in fighting and preventing cancer, many citrus fruits from oranges and grapefruits to tangerines are often credited with anti-allergy attributes, improving blood flow, while reducing and preventing inflammation.

To the great benefit of humanity, the widespread abundance of separate flavonoid-packed plants is so vast that to list them all comprehensively and abundantly would take several volumes of printed books or hundreds of Web pages. By some estimates, at least 5,000 separate plant species contain flavonoids

Those of us determined to achieve or maintain good health need to take a continual and aggressive role in adding flavonoids to our diets. You see, despite their abundance, these foods are not generally contained within most typical meal plans.

That's why patients and consumers everywhere should actively seek flavonoid drinks and foods at restaurants or when grocery shopping.

Chapter 18 Summary

People striving to prevent cancer and those being treated for the disease should eat lots of antioxidant foods that help eliminate toxins and free radicals that cause tumors. Many of these invaders enter the body via food consumption, while other carcinogens occur in the environment around us. The need for eating antioxidant foods has intensified in recent decades due to the spread of dangerous chemicals in the environment, plus the advent of preservatives included in the food packaging and preserving processes. Dangerous food-preparation methods also cause free radicals, such as overcooking red meat on grills. Naturally occurring foods high in flavonoids and vitamins are often excellent anti-carcinogens. One of the most potent flavonoids is low-sugar dark chocolate. Additional foods or herbs with high-flavonoid content include sea buckthorn, white tea, red onions, barriers, ginkgo biloba, and red wine. Many citrus fruits also are packed with anti-carcinogen attributes.

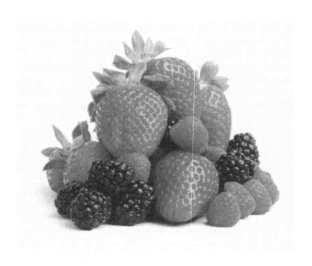

Chapter 19

Use Antioxidants
as Formidable Weapons

Besides adding flavonoids to their good-health strategies, cancer patients also need to employ healthy doses of additional foods listed as "antioxidants." Of course, rather than taking matters into your own hands, such an overall lifestyle strategy should only be launched under the careful guidance of a health care professional or a dietitian.

Before actively getting massive quantities of antioxidants, you need to know that these are supplements or foods that counteract, prevent or minimize the harmful effects of free radicals. As you might recall, free radicals are atoms that have not attached to or bonded with other atoms. Unless the killer T-cell system successfully removes or destroys such invaders, these usurpers can damage your DNA's biological map—ultimately resulting in tumors.

Great care should be taken in the process of ingesting adequate healthful amounts of antioxidants. Like the over-ingestion of almost any substance, eating far too many antioxidants in one sitting—massive amounts of foods or supplements—can result in medical complications. For instance, many people might not realize this, but drinking far too much water at an excessively high rate within a short period can lead to organ failure or even death. The same goes for the over-consumption of certain minerals such as iron, shown as a precursor to potential increases in the risk of breast cancer and other cancers when ingested at dangerous, unnaturally high levels.

Moderation at a consistent and healthful rate can serve as the key to success in using antioxidants to battle cancer. Luckily from the perspective of patients with this disease, natural antioxidant foods grow in relative abundance both in wild-land areas and as crops.

Throughout the animal world and within the plant kingdom the need for antioxidants is so essential that many organisms make them naturally for their own protection. Among just some of the most prevalent antioxidants made in nature:

Vitamin C

Considered essential for human life, serving many vital functions and particularly its critical role as an antioxidant, Vitamin C helps to eliminate or control free radicals. On a molecular and biological level, from the lay person's view Vitamin C performs complex functions that generate numerous important reactions with the body's enzymes.

A person who ingests inadequate amounts of Vitamin C risks the possibility of scurvy, a serious medical condition. A lack of Vitamin C robs the body of its ability to synthesize collagen, resulting in many debilitating symptoms like spongy gums, spots on the thighs and legs, and a pale appearance—plus in advanced stages the loss of teeth, neuropathy, jaundice, fever and even death.

Animals rarely or never suffer from scurvy because unlike humans their bodies internally produce Vitamin C. The incidence of scurvy on a worldwide scale sharply decreased after 1932 when researchers determined the cause of the disease, which wasn't known until then.

Before this discovery, people who stayed away from land for extended periods—particularly pirates and ocean-crossing vessels—often suffered from scurvy. Through the early 1900s and particularly hundreds of years ago, shipmates in the British Navy got the name "limies" when the cause of their disease was cured by limes. Within foods, Vitamin C can be found in a wide variety of crops and even meats in extremely small amounts, but it is most commonly found in fruits, especially citrus varieties.

Of the 40 most frequently listed plant sources for Vitamin C, the species with by far the highest milligram content of this essential substance is the Kakadu plum. Just one of these fruits has from 1,000 milligrams to 5,300 milligrams of Vitamin C. This compares to 50 milligrams in oranges. Also known as "billy goat plum" and "gubinge" from a flowering plant abundant in the Arnhem Land of east Australia, slim and medium-size trees that grow Kakadu plum average more than 65 feet tall. Possibly first enjoyed in abundance by native Australian Aborigines, Kakadu plums were primarily sold until recently for industrial purposes.

As news of its potency spread in recent decades businesses started using this amazing fruit as a food supplement and to boost Vitamin C levels in juice. Sadly, high demand led some people to prematurely harvest the fruit in quantities exceeding government-capped levels.

Coming in second place on the Vitamin C content charts compiled from a variety of sources is "camo-camo," a riverside tree found most frequently in the Amazon rainforests of Peru, at 2,800 milligrams.

Also growing naturally in such diverse South American

nations as Brazil, Bolivia, Colombia and Equador, camo-camo is more readily available in international markets than Kakadu plum. Within the broad spectrum of Vitamin-C laden foods, acerola and Sea-buckthorn come in third and fourth place with 1,677 milligrams and 695 milligrams respectively.

Vitamin E

Although among the most powerful antioxidants, Vitamin E might be overlooked by many people seeking anti-cancer benefits.

This oversight happens at least on occasion because many of the most recent sources of Vitamin E come from foods that some consumers might unwittingly strive to ignore when dieting. Along with salad dressing, other frequent sources are corn oil and soybean oil. On a molecular level, Vitamin E is often associated with:

Tocopherols: In its "alpha form," this class of chemical compounds if found more frequently in European diets in foods like sunflower seeds and olive oil, and in its "gamma form" more common in American diets from corn oil and soybean.

Tocotrienols: Besides working to prevent cancer, this segment strives to strengthen brain cells and to reduce cholesterol. The antioxidant attributes of tocotrienols are deemed by scientists as more powerful than tocopherols due to a unique side chain with the atomic structure of this class, enabling it to better penetrate fatty layers of the liver and brain.

Adding to these benefits, according to a 2009 report in "Nutrition and Cancer," tocotrienols can lower tumor formation, while lessening cell damage and protecting DNA. Additional good news spread in the 1990s on results of studies indicating tocotrienol minimizes the incidence of breast cancer growth in humans.

More reason for optimism spread in 1997 when the "Journal of Nutrition" reported that a commonly used breast cancer medication worked well with tocotrienol.

Increasing the reputation of this classification even more, an additional study indicated that in gamma form tocotrienol targets a key cancer-promoting protein, Id1, killing the disease's cells and preventing their spread. This became especially good news to people with melanoma or prostate cancer.

Besides being available in supplement form under a health care professional's supervision, the tocotrienol form can be found in: rice; the fruit of palm trees from temperate, tropical and subtropical climates; and annatto, derived from seeds of achiote trees grown only in tropical and subtropical regions.

When produced commercially, annatto is often used as a food coloring, particularly for many types of cheese such as Red Leicester, Glouchester and cheddar, for a wide variety of cheese-based products, and within dairy spreads like butter and margarine.

In addition, annatto is sometimes used as a flavor enhancer in Caribbean and Latin American meals, heralded for a sweet, peppery and slightly nutty taste. Despite the widespread use of annatto, patient's need a health professional's guidance because this spice or coloring may cause rare allergic reactions.

Resveratrol

Within the class of polyphenolic antioxidants, these contain everything from the spices oregano and cinnamon to chocolate, to various fruits, olive oil, soy, coffee and tea.

A variety of fungi and bacteria pathogens produce this stilbenoid and phytoalexin. A type of natural phenol, the stilbenoid aspect is often found in grapes considered by scientists to have many health benefits.

The phytoalexin segment is believed to serve significant antioxidant protections by attacking invasive organisms by puncturing cell walls. This can help prevent cancer cells from maturing, seriously disrupting the disease's metabolism and stifling a tumor's ability to grow or spread.

Through evolution, certain plants have naturally developed resveratrol as a protective mechanism. Besides grapes, it's derived from numerous plants including the smallanthus fruticosus, rice, carrots and papaya fruit.

Some researchers believe that besides its anti-cancer action, this food also can lower cholesterol, help cardiovascular functions, and prevent inflammation. Many scientists also proclaim that the skin of red grapes is among the most significant sources, heralded as having significant anti-aging attributes.

In laboratory and commercial venues, scientists are able to create bioengineered microorganisms mimicking resveratrol for distribution as a nutritional supplement.

According to some reports, Japanese knotweed has been used for this production process. But the "Los Angeles Times" and a National Academy of Science publication have quoted researchers as saying they do not know the long-term effectiveness of such supplements.

Besides its antioxidant attributes, resveratrol may possess significant anti-aging power by lengthening telomeres.

In 2006, "Current Biology" reported that in Italy scientists in laboratory tests were able to use resveratrol to increase by 56 percent the lifespan of a species fish that typically live only nine weeks. Some scientists theorize that a weak toxic action that resveratrol generates ultimately sparks an organism's defense mechanisms into overdrive and thus extending life. Meantime, the significant effect—if any—of resveratrol on cancer in humans remains controversial as research and testing continue.

A vast range of other research indicates that resveratrol naturally and efficiently declares all-out war on esophageal tumors and cancers within the intestinal tract. Potentially deadly skin melanomas also can get obliterated when used as a topical application, reportedly because reveratrol seizes opportune chances to protect the skin from current or potential damage caused by dangerous UVB exposure—ultraviolet radiation.

Even so, at least according to some studies reveratrol should never be considered a "cure-all" impacting all forms of cancer. As reported by various nutritional and pharmacological publications, in several tests it had no effect when given orally to patients suffering from lung cancer or leukemia.

Conversely, other reports showed that when administered to mice by injection resveratrol slowed the metastatic growth of Lewis lung carcinomas.

Additional research on animals indicates that resveratrol has no impact on existing mammary tumors, although this substance appeared to prevent such disease, as recorded in various publications.

Although acknowledging the many positive attributes of resveratrol, some doctors might urge pregnant women to avoid this substance. A 2010 report in the "Cancer Letter" and a 2006 article in a journal of food chemistry said resveratrol mirrors the effects of certain anti-cancer drugs. However, the natural characteristics within resveratrol are sometimes thought to have anticarcinogenic and carcinogenic attributes in certain circumstances, particularly instances involving the human fetus. When in the womb, unborn babies might be negatively susceptible to resveratrol's strength because in that stage of growth humans lack some ability to process toxins.

Besides the skin of grapes, resveratrol has been found in the roots of the Japanese knotweed. The amounts found in grape skin can vary depending on species and where plants grow. Many wine aficionados like to brag that their favorite drink contains this extremely healthy substance, which also can help cardiovascular functions.

The amounts and potency of resveratrol in different wines also varies, partly hinged on the duration and processes used in the fermentation process of production. Vineyards usually produce red wine with skins, while white wine producers usually remove this portion. Some reports claim that both white and red wines made with muscadine grapes contain higher concentrations of resveratrol.. But various studies give conflicting conclusions.

While most media reports focus solely on the benefits of resveratrol derived from grapes, a 2005 journal on agricultural food chemistry claims that peanuts—especially sprouted varieties—have high levels of this substance, equaling or surpassing the amounts typically found in grapes.

Adding to the mix, some health food companies sell mulberry fruit, and especially the skin from such plants, touted as nutritional supplements containing resveratrol. Also failing to get as much positive media attention is dark chocolate, plus baking chocolate and cocoa powder.

Thanks largely to widespread positive publicity regarding resveratrol since the start of the 21st Century, streams of news reports in recent years have chronicled great sales increases of this substance in supplement form. However, as acknowledged in various news stories, the effective amounts of resveratrol in differing supplements can vary. For this reason, I recommend that consumers and patients only seek resveratrol in supplement form when referred directly, in person by an experienced medial professional—especially a naturopath, homeopath or a professional with a PhD in nutrition.

Carotenoids

Also potentially powerful antioxidants, carotenoids occur naturally within the cells of plants. Some capture light energy for storage as molecules for use in the process of transforming this sun-given power for its own use. This photosynthesis ultimately serves as the source of energy for all life on Earth. Within the carotenoid segment, this is handled by the chloroplast segment.

The second segment is covered by chromoplasts that generate pigment for plants, and for storage with unique organisms where membranes are enclosed around complex structures. Chromoplasts are often found within aging or stressed leaves, roots, certain fruit species, and specific flowers.

In the form of Vitamin A, humans process or generate activity involving four different types of carotenoids:

Beta-Carotene: Abundant in many plants and fruits, this bright-colored orange and reddish pigment is a hydrocarbon and important organic compound important for processing 40 carbons via eight units of isoprene—a relatively common organic compound. As distinguished from the three other types within the carotenoid category, beta-carotene has distinctive rings at both ends of its molecules. These are among attributes that give carrots their orange color. The strength of this characteristic motivates some manufacturers to isolate carotenoid material for use as food coloring. Besides also serving as a primary worldwide source for Vitamin A, the active ingredients in beta-carotene serve an important process in helping the body absorb the important antioxidant attributes within Vitamin E. Like other types within the carotenoid class, the body's ability to absorb and use beta-carotene depends on the healthy function of the duodenum within the small intestine. In addition, the body's ultimate ability to process beta-carotene depends on the effectiveness of what scientists call the "scavenger receptor" within a class called B1. Thus, in order for your body to benefit from this potentially powerful antioxidant, certain intricate cellular processes must work efficiently. Largely due to this reason, especially for cancer patients I cannot begin to stress the importance of taking the essential measures needed to maintain a healthy gut as described earlier. According to some scientific research, even in healthy people the body's ability to absorb and use beta-carotene is only from 9 percent to 22 percent. Rather than just carrots, beta-carotene generates the orange color in a variety of vegetables and fruits. The most well-known fruits include papayas, mangoes, and cantaloupe. Besides carrots, yams are among other root vegetables containing beta-carotene. People seeking to benefit from this powerful category should remember that beta-carotene also is contained in numerous green vegetables such as sweet potato leaves, spinach, kale, sweet gourd leaves and leafy vegetables. Some sources indicate that among all fruits and vegetables the foods with the greatest beta-carotene content are crude palm oil and Vietnamese gac, a fruit also found in southeast China and northeast Australia. Other beta-carotene food sources include sweet potatoes, pumpkins and collards. Some homeopaths and dietitians warn patients that people who eat huge quantities of foods containing beta-carotene sometimes get orange-tinged skin, a condition called "carotenemia." In addition, although beta-carotene is a natural food with strong antioxidant qualities you should only take large amounts under a medical professional's supervision. This is because, according to a "Medicine Plus" report, extremely high doses of beta-carotene in supplement form can lead to lung cancer among patients who smoke. This study has not been verified. Some researchers also worry about the possibility that supplements of beta-carotene might lower the life expectancy of people who smoke, cause cardiovascular problems, generate brain hemorrhages or even form prostate cancer. In addition, beta-carotene can counteract medications taken to control cholesterol, minimizing or eliminating the effectiveness of those drugs. In addition, doctors urge people who take a weight-loss drug, Orlistat, to reduce their consumption of beta-carotene by about one third. According to a U.S. government publication distributed in May 2012, people who eat beta-carotene while drinking alcohol sometimes develop hepatotoxicity—commonly called "liver damage," after those drinks decrease the ability of their bodies to convert beta-carotene into Vitamin A—called "retinol" within the body. Largely for these reasons, as a medical professional fighting cancer, I sometimes urge patients to get most of their beta-carotene primarily from natural food sources rather than via supplements, and also to ingest large amounts of this natural substance only when under the advice of a medical professional. In addition, patients need to clearly understand that although vast numbers of homeopaths, health professionals and scientists generally consider beta-carotene as a powerful antioxidant for preventing cancer, the effectiveness of its apparent ability to treat existing tumors remains an issue. A report by the American Cancer Society on Vitamin A and carotenoids says their ability to treat and to prevent cancer is not proven. However, studies in head and neck cancers are ongoing.

Alpha-carotene: As one of the four segments within the carotenoid sector, this form has molecules with one ring at each end. Like beta-carotene, yellow-orange vegetables within this segment include sweet potatoes, pumpkins and carrots. Alpha-carotene also is contained within certain dark green vegetables, particularly leaf lettuce, green peas, broccoli and green beans. These can serve as powerful antioxidants, possessing positive anti-cancer attributes.

Gamma-carotene: Unlike beta-carotene and alpha-carotene, which can be produced biologically within the bodies of many animals, gamma-carotene can only be generated within plants. Many of the same foods that naturally have beta-carotene and alpha-carotene also produce gamma-carotene. These generally range from carrots and sweet potatoes to cantaloupe. The bodies of some plant-eating animals do a relatively poor job of converting carotenoid characteristics into colorless retinoid substances. For instance, chickens and even humans who lack effective biological methods of processing gamma-carotene sometimes accumulate a yellow tinge in their own body fat. On the positive side, gamma-carotene is contained within a large number of plants, various species that do not contain the beta-carotene and alpha-carotene antioxidants. Gamma-carotene is within some of the same plants, like carrots, sweet potatoes, mangoes and pumpkins. It's also in cassava, rose hips, ivy gourd, romaine lettuce, parsley, watercress, mustard greens, persimmon and apricots. Some food experts insist that the human body does a better job absorbing gamma-carotene while the individual also ingests fats. This becomes possible because gamma-carotene is fat soluble. As with all natural foods, gamma-carotene can potentially generate health problems when ingested in abnormally high quantities. For all carotene classes, scientists call adverse physical reactions from the over-ingestion of carotene "carotenemia" or "hypercarotenemia." Carotene is non-toxic, whereas excessive amounts of Vitamin A—although not considered dangerous—can cause skin to have an orange tinge. This spares the conjunctiva.

Cryptoxanthin: Prevalent in apples, egg yolks, butter, orange rinds and papaya, this class of carotene has a red crystalline solid. Like the other carotenes, cryptoxanthin converts to Vitamin A when within the human body—while also performing a vital chore as an antioxidant in battling free radicals, preventing cell damage and protecting DNA. Cryptoxanthin has been shown by the results of several epidemiological studies as reducing the risk of lung cancer, according to a 2006 report by the International Journal of Cancer. Other studies on the effect of cryptoxathin on patients with malignant cancers of the brain or the spine gave less promising results, generating "poorer survival" when ingested in moderate or high amounts.

Chapter 19 Summary

Many powerful antioxidant foods grow in nature, helpful in assisting the body's various types of protective cells in preventing or fighting cancer. Among the most powerful are Vitamin C and Vitamin E. Vitamin C is abundant in many citrus fruits, and Vitamin E is abundant in numerous food sources including rice, the fruit of palm trees and annatto, derived from seeds of achiote trees. Another powerful antioxidant is Resveratrol, often found in the skin of grapes, plus wines, grape juice, peanuts and lower amounts in cocoa powder. Another powerful antioxidant food sector is carotenoids. The beta-carotene foods within this class include vegetables, fruits, carrots, yams, sweet potato leaves, spinach, sweet gourd leaves, leafy vegetables and Vietnamese gac, a fruit from Southeast Asia and Australia. Foods from the alpha-carotene segment within the carotenoid class include dark leafy vegetables, sweet potatoes, pumpkins, carrots, green peas, green beans and broccoli. Foods from the two remaining carotenoid sectors, gamma-carotene and cryptoxanthin, include sweet potatoes, mangoes, pumpkins, apples, egg yolks, butter, orange rinds and papaya.

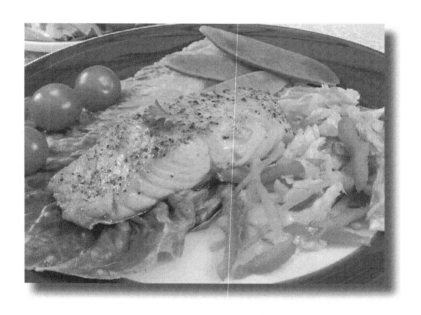

Chapter 20

Antioxidants
Assist Vital Liver Function

Patients eating antioxidants in hopes of preventing or controlling cancers should know that many of these beneficial effects benefit the liver. As you've already learned, that essential organ performs key filtering and processing functions critical to life.

Patients and consumers who already have worked to cleanse their livers, gallbladders and intestines can position themselves to optimize potential benefits from antioxidants. Among the many specific functions when this happens:

Break: While the liver already works non-stop to eliminate or process metals ranging from iron to zinc, antioxidants can break up such substances when they have elements that have incomplete atoms that could otherwise harm cells and damage DNA.

Empower: Simultaneously, antioxidants often clear the way for potential benefits from metals that sometimes serve as "antioxidant nutrients" like zinc and selenium. On their own, these elements lack antioxidant attributes. Yet these chemical elements help to enable antioxidant enzymes to protect the body.

Uric Acid Plays an Essential Role

Scientists also universally agree that within humans, uric acid serves a critical and essential role as a powerful and necessary antioxidant. Yet its effectiveness in addressing diseases like multiple sclerosis and cancer remains controversial.

Uric acid also can damage health when accumulating within the body in excessive amounts. One of the most common negative outcomes is gout, a form of arthritis, or other medical complications like diabetes and kidney stones.

Despite these occasional drawbacks uric acid may play a role as an important antioxidant, according to a 2005 article in "Current Pharmaceutical Design." Even so, various medical papers and articles published during the past few decades indicate scientists still lack definitive answers on whether uric acid prevents or causes stroke or the hardening of arteries.

Conversely, low levels of uric acid can lead to anemia. Some researchers might suspect that contraceptives pull down uric acid levels in some women, although I have yet to find any conclusive reports on this theory.

Within humans, uric acid is formed within the body when certain enzymes break down. In healthy individuals the urination process removes excess amounts from the body. Problems within this process can damage the liver or kidneys.

A person's propensity to generate excessive amounts of uric acid also might result from genetics, inheriting such propensities from ancestors.

Among cancer patients, the need to achieve optimal levels of uric acid becomes critical. Too much of this substance could result in medical complications that complicate the person's overall treatment regimen. So, patients should take a pro-active role in taking these steps:

188

Checkup: Ask your doctor to review your uric acid levels within your blood tests.

Meals: Especially if the exam indicates your body has excessive amounts of uric acid, you should avoid foods suspected of elevating the substance like rich foods containing "purines." Eating foods containing too much table sugar has been listed as a potential cause in various medical journals. Some physicians and researchers also cite rapid weight loss or fasting as a potential cause, with the body elevating uric acid levels as a protective action.

Food types: Reports vary on which foods tend to elevate uric acid. Besides sardines and the liver of animals, other foods that some dietitians recommend avoiding in excessive quantities: fish, seafood, asparagus, oatmeal, green peas, mushrooms, wheat bran, wheat germ, pork and beef. Many of the foods rich in flavonoid, especially some fruits such as those already listed, contain fructose or sugars that in turn increase the body's synthesis of the antioxidant uric acid. A rapid killing off of cancer by chemotherapy can cause acute gout due to high levels of uric acid.

The Good Mixes with the Bad

A paradoxical situation arises when some physicians insist specific foods are "good" while other doctors swear those same meals are definitely "bad."

Some foods that many health professionals say to avoid in order to prevent too much uric acid are simultaneously touted as having strong antioxidant, anti-cancer attributes

For instance, you might recall that asparagus and green peas are among foods listed as having ideal levels of carotene antioxidants, while fruits high in flavonoid often get similar praise. But those same foods also are sometimes considered unhealthful among those eager to lower or minimize uric acid.

The overall situation of conflicting medical studies sometimes becomes so pathetic that consumers occasionally do not know whether to laugh or cry. Some news stories, for instance, have championed coffee for its supposedly undeniable anti-cancer attributes, while other reports seem to indicate that java lacks significant antioxidant qualities.

The same goes for the consumption of red meats, which I personally believe based on experience and various research reports has predominantly unhealthful qualities. In a world-famous court case, beef producers sued media superstar Oprah Winfrey for publicly questioning the healthfulness of eating their products.

Even so, I tell my patients—especially those over age 50—to avoid eating red meats or to at least limit such meals to several times each year at most. While studies seem to sharply conflict on this issue, I personally believe that excessive consumption of red, non-poultry meat among some people could be a key trigger in causing cancers.

Despite what avid vegetarians might tell us, meat is a primary source of iron for people across many cultures. Without adequate iron, people often develop serious overall physical weakness called "anemia." To counteract or to prevent this potential problem, some anti-cancer diets might include high-protein poultry or fish.

Compounding these various overall challenges, many scientists agree that almost all foods contain "anti-nutrient" attributes. Such propensities interfere with the person's natural ability to adequately absorb and process nutrients, essential for good health. A 2006 article in "Oxford University Press" said that anti-nutrients are natural and synthetic compounds. Once again we're faced with an issue integral to cancer patients. Among these many instances are situations where phytic acid—which stores phosphorous in many plants—blocks the body's ability to absorb minerals like copper, iron, zinc and calcium, by forming insoluble complexes that impede the process. A Cornell University project has concluded that due to a variety of factors almost all foods contain at least some anti-nutrients.

Largely for these reasons, from my view, dietary supplements designed to increase the body's ingestion of crucial vitamins and minerals should be considered for almost every well-rounded anti-cancer diet regimen, and for use during treatment of the disease when approved by a physician.

Accept the Controversies

As a cancer patient or even as a typical consumer, you need to acknowledge the fact that doctors and researchers often disagree on the supposed effectiveness of certain foods in preventing or managing cancer.

Ultimately, you'll be the person making these choices for yourself. Except for those in hospital or nursing home environments where management dictates much of the menu, each consumer or cancer patient makes his or her own decision regarding what to eat and how much.

You need to take a pro-active mode, rather than allowing the massive amounts of conflicting data on the supposed health benefits or dangers of foods to cause confusion.

To do this, as I often tell patients, "you should learn as much as you can about these issues, and eventually choose the foods that you consider ideal for your particular medical challenges and needs."

Upon learning the many benefits of antioxidant foods, many people become mystified and increasingly curious upon discovering that our bodies also naturally produce a wide variety of anti-carcinogens.

Chapter 20 Summary

Antioxidant foods fortify liver function, enabling the organ to break down and remove potentially harmful meals including excessively high concentrations of iron and zinc. These same foods also help the liver make the best use of metals including zinc and selenium that help protect the body from cancer. Uric acid from foods like fish, seafood and asparagus also can serve as a helpful antioxidant. But low levels of uric acid can lead to health problems like anemia. Also, too much of this substance can cause medical problems like gout, or problems with the kidneys and liver. Patients should seek continuous advice from homeopaths or dietitians, partly because some natural foods deemed as antioxidants also can generate health problems under specific conditions.

Chapter 21

Diet Challenges Before and During Chemotherapy

Diet challenges sometimes become formidable for cancer patients as they undergo chemotherapy, which often damages their digestive systems while depleting the body's essential natural bone marrow and often resulting in extensive hair loss.

As many patients already know beforehand, high-dose chemotherapy contains one or more poisons designed to attack and destroy cancer. But the treatments often destroy good, otherwise healthy cells in the process.

Particularly when administered in high doses, chemotherapy treatment sometimes kills or severely damages critical organs—often resulting in the patient's death.

Remember, this is among primary reasons why I became a homeopath, expanding services so that I could offer more natural, non-poisonous lower-dose remedies rather than just practice conventional oncology.

I've helped many patients who had begun to "waste away" when previously under the care of standard-medicine doctors elsewhere. While under my care, the vast majority of my patients choose treatments other than standard, high-dose chemotherapy, and have better survival rates.

Wasting Away

Efforts to assist stage IV cancer patients who have lost extensive weight become formidable, because without good nutrition even healthy people fail to maintain their vibrancy for very long. These hurdles can become particularly challenging, especially among patients who become extremely weak upon losing extensive body weight. Remember, all cancer diets are weight-loss diets.

The wide variety of potential gastrointestinal symptoms can range from constipation and diarrhea to vomiting and debilitating nausea. These conditions in turn can lead to severe malnutrition, robbing the body of some or all of its natural abilities to fight cancer. Along with dehydration, these symptoms sometimes result at least partly from the failure to eat or drink enough during treatments, or to hold down foods for extended periods. When this happens on occasion a patient becomes steadily weaker physically, creating a cascading effect that can lead to critical illness.

Worsening matters, even before reaching that urgent stage, the nausea and periodic vomiting sometimes generate gastrointestinal damage. All these various adverse symptoms invariably increase the overall challenges faced by the patient and his or her physicians.

Good Nutrition is the Key

The key to eventual recovery amid chemotherapy hinges on good, sound nutrition coupled with positive efforts to maintain or to repair the digestive system.

Every person undergoing this phase, no matter how

challenging the situation needs to remember this resounding message loud and clear: "Your body wants to live. Every cell of your body yearns for itself and for your entire organism to remain alive. As long as you are breathing and conscious, no matter how much pain you're currently enduring, until such time as your body gives a final shut-off signal to itself—most likely while you're unconscious—you need to consciously give yourself a fighting chance."

Yes, rather than merely just eating as much nutritious food as you can to bolster the digestive system, a positive attitude reigns as a formidable key in leading to your eventual recovery.

Indeed, without a positive, "can-do" perspective some patients who have already suffered extensive nausea, digestive problems and weight loss, will discover that their attempts to get well seem insurmountable.

Relatives, Friends and Professionals

When and if you reach such a serious stage within your cancer treatment and recovery process, the assistance, guidance and support of the healthy people around you becomes critical. Even patients who feel "alone" without friends or supportive relatives can often find courage and mental strength thanks to support from medical professionals.

Cancer patients who get occasional or even non-stop support from family members or acquaintances can feel doubly lucky. Many people with cancer including lots of mature persons are not as fortunate.

Now in the fifth decade of my career as a medical professional, I have witnessed thousands of instances where positive attitudes increase the probability of recovery—a perspective embraced by most people with cancer. Patients that become emotionally depressed, giving up far too early, position themselves to die far too soon.

Stressing the importance of such an attitude might seem far too easy to verbalize, or to write in a book when the messenger is not the person who has to physically suffer.

So, how do you feel positive at the very moment that you're experiencing nausea and vomiting during or after chemotherapy? What can and should you tell yourself, when and if eventually suffering extensive digestive and gastrointestinal problems?

The answer, I urge patients to tell themselves is this, "The necessary key to my eventual good health is to eat well." Even among many seriously ill people, this critical task can become possible thanks to advances in medical technology. Lots of patients have endured the same retching, painful conditions that you might be suffering from now, and they fully recovered to enjoy many years in good health. For any of this to eventually happen, chemo patients need to eat the recommended foods as regularly and consistently as possible. And, if they're unable to do that now, a team of medical professionals has the ability, technology and strategies to help put your health back on a positive path.

When Thinking Becomes "Fuzzy"

For some patients, fatigue caused by continually debilitating and ultimately painful chemo can lead to mental depression. Rest assured that when and if such symptoms kick into gear, you'll be surrounded by medical professionals who know how to address such issues as they erupt. Ideally, you and these experts should share various goals, especially getting you onto a pathway toward good, continuous nutrition. Among just some of the primary hurdles that could lead to weakness and a loss of appetite, and ways to address them:

Fatigue: The ongoing and seemingly endless fight against cancer and particularly the adverse symptoms of chemotherapy can leave the patient exhausted—both physically and emotionally. This, in turn, can result in a loss of interest in food, a doorway to worsening overall health. A common result of malignancy is anemia, severe weakness not always due to inadequate levels of iron in the blood. The anemic condition robs the body of its ability to intake adequate amounts of oxygen, sometimes leading to difficulty in breathing and even struggles to walk. If this happens to you amid chemo, seriously consider taking your doctor's advice if the physician recommends a blood transfusion, or taking iron, Vitamin B12 or folic acid. This treatment alone sometimes sharply boosts energy and begins reversing anemia within a relatively short period, clearing the way for the resumption of a healthy appetite.

Weakened immunity: Chemo causes widespread and pervasive cell damage throughout the body, particularly when administered in high doses. This can wreak havoc on your body's critical immune systems—essential for maintaining good health, and for enjoying the benefits of a healthy appetite. Cancer patients socked with this condition face potentially formidable challenges, since immune deficiencies can make eating extremely difficult. At least according to some publications, a whopping 85 percent of infections among chemo patients occur even in cases where they've followed the medical professionals' advice on how to avoid becoming ill, and the need to wash their hands often. Severe infections, particularly within a patient's gastrointestinal tract—even inside the mouth or on the skin—can lead to sepsis, a potentially deadly condition where vital organs throughout the body reach an inflammatory state. So, if you undergo chemotherapy, be sure to follow your medical team's instructions about cleanliness and crowds, continually mindful that your immune system needs to remain as strong as possible so that you can eat and get well.

Bleeding: Some chemo rids the body of vital platelets that protect your body from excessive bleeding. When platelets drop to critically low levels of less than 50,000, the patient faces the danger of potentially serious bleeding if cut or from extensive, unsightly bruises. Having the precarious condition of a low platelet count also might hinder your ability to ingest and absorb enough nutrition to fully recover. Primarily for these reasons, some physicians choose to postpone chemotherapy amid the treatment schedule if the platelet count dips too low. If this happens to you, follow the physicians' or dietitians' meal and snack selections in order to keep your body as strong as possible—increasing the probability for full recovery. Also, avoid blood-thinning supplements like aspirin, Vitamin E, ginkgo biloba, omega-3 fatty acids and ginseng.

Digestive issues: These are among the most frequent, predictable problems suffered by chemo patients. While many people experience extreme, potentially debilitating weight loss, a small percentage actually gain pounds when they overeat in hopes of blocking the symptoms of heartburn or even nausea. Determined to effectively address these negative symptoms beforehand or at the onset of issues, some physicians administer "anti-emetic" drugs to handle nausea and vomiting. Although some doctors might strongly urge this route in all instances, I prescribe such medications only when deemed necessary. That's because a primary goal should be enabling the patient to maintain a natural, healthy appetite whenever possible. Potential adverse side effects from anti-emetic medications include motion sickness, sedation and dry mouth, particularly those from the opioid or "opium" class of analgesics, produced from the same substance used to make heroin.

Complications can Hamper Diets

Only a small percentage of my patients choose high-dose chemotherapy. Remember that as an oncologist, I must give all of them that option.

As already stated, my clinic offers a variety of cancer treatments that sometimes feature what doctors list as "low-dose" treatments. Occasionally when that happens, or even when no chemo drugs are given all, a patient sometimes suffers from complications.

Largely for this reason, I often suggest that people treated at my clinic enjoy their recommended foods throughout the day—even in small quantities. Remember that our bodies are slow-burning fuel mechanisms. Our bodies use and process the foods that we've eaten for use as energy. This is remarkable partly because although separate meals can last for extended periods, the actual phases of swallowing food takes less than several minutes collectively throughout the entire day. In this sense, your stomach serves as your initial fuel tank.

On a basic, primary level, at least for descriptive purposes this short-term storage process is the equivalent to the gas tank in a car. For healthy people and particularly individuals with cancer, continued operation of the body depends fully on its efficiency in conducting this slow fuel-burning process.

Here's where the food-as-fuel concept becomes particularly critical for cancer patients. To put this into a clear, easy-to-understand perspective, think of how an efficient, fast-moving car operates. Placing your foot on the accelerator sends miniscule amounts of gasoline into the engine, where the fuel ignites—

generating enough energy to turn pistons to make the wheels turn. When your car moves, miniature, continuous and rapid-fire explosions occur non-stop. In a finely-tuned, efficient car the necessary explosions cannot happen without oxygen. Lubricants and coolants keep the parts flowing with ease. Without all these various processes the car shuts down, particularly if the fuel source gets blocked. When the car is working fine, and when the fuel gets used and spent, the byproduct gets pushed out of the tailpipe as CO and CO2.

Well, in a basic mechanical sense confined to biology and not metallurgy, this is what happens for your body. This comparison often helps put the situation into perspective for patients who lack a clear understanding of biology.

Particularly among people with cancer, but also for healthy individuals, food serves as the fuel to run their entire bodies. Within the body, the internal combustion engine that comes in the form of the lungs for accepting critical oxygen, the heart for transporting energy and digestive system all serve as your most critical engine parts.

Pay Attention to Your Food

When anything goes terribly wrong, dipping to extremely critical levels, within any of these vital functions the patient could die. A lack of proper oxygen, nutrients or insufficient amounts of antioxidants can damage the body's internal processes, where a wide variety of complexes depend greatly on each other.

A good-functioning interaction between all organs is essential for healthy people. With even greater urgency, a person with stage IV cancer or advancing levels of the disease becomes particularly susceptible to potential complications. Often when that happens, the disease can cause specific necessary organs or internal

200

functions to go haywire.

This is largely why cancer patients can potentially improve their probability for recovery by digesting healthy foods and nutrients on a continuous basis. Especially for them, this does not mean eating good meals once every blue moon or striving to gouge themselves with all the right servings in a single sitting.

To get a clear focus of the issue, think of this. You would not want all the fuel in your car to explode all at once. Such an occurrence would cause catastrophic results for your body. When over-eating unhealthy foods, the stomach and intestines can go haywire, striving too hard to perform difficult tasks. Such situations, in turn, could cause the creation of free radicals that go unchecked, resulting in cancer growth and metastasis

You Need Energy

Ultimately, everything comes down to this for cancer patients as far as diet: "You need to have continual physical energy provided by well-absorbed nutrients from food, in order to survive, recover and to thrive."

Regaining and maintaining good health will become possible only if you steadily push only adequate amounts of the necessary energy made possible by food into your body—in much the same way that an efficient car expends fuel as the vehicle glides down a highway as if butter atop a grill.

For the most part, this means that your body needs continuous, regularly scheduled, and relatively small consistent shots of energy, largely in order to maintain the vibrancy required to successfully prevent, manage or control its cancer. Certainly eating only a healthy breakfast early in the morning and a fair dinner late at night in a single day could leave you feeling sluggish and tired at mid-day.

Because the body needs energy to thrive and to survive, such a mid-day lethargic condition could leave you susceptible to the ravages of cancer and various complications from the disease. Indeed, skipping meals, eating too light or going far longer than necessary without adequate amounts of food is essentially the equivalent to "letting your body stall smack-dab in the middle of the big proverbial freeway that we call life. When that happens, cancer can crash into you with horrific speed, ferocious and uncaring."

Some of the proverbial "cars" zipping past you, and potentially deeper into your organism, include the very free radicals and cancers that you're trying to resist. The potential danger heightens and intensifies among cancer patients who either refuse to or fail to refuel their body's internal fuel tank with sufficient energy throughout the day.

Focus on Recovery

Some of these eating challenges among cancer patients occur because their doctors—usually standard-medicine oncologists—fail to explain the significance of eating consistent and regular amounts of recommended foods.

In fact, I would argue that a vast majority of oncologists barely mention the subject of meals or they fail to talk about this critical subject altogether.

From my perspective, the daily obituary pages are filled with many people who would still be alive if they had been given an opportunity to learn and to understand the vital significance of continuously eating small, efficient and vitamin-packed amounts of recommended foods. When writing of these obits notifying the public of their loved one's death, many grieving relatives proclaim that he or she "fought a courageous battle against cancer." Much of the time when that happens, I believe, the deceased person suffered far too much—more than necessary, in many instances perhaps due to inadequate eating regimens.

Of course, eating right should not be considered the "be-all, and end-all" singular factor in attempts to prevent, control or effectively manage cancer. Yet what the general public considers as "recovery" can never become possible for these people without consistent and adequate nutrition.

Appreciate Food from the Start

Even if they have already received treatment elsewhere for their current cancers, when people enter my clinic for the first time they soon learn that our recommended foods have become a top priority in their treatment regimens.

Understandably, many patients soon tell me that they're surprised by this. In essence, they're saying: "I didn't know any of this until now. I'm stunned that my previous doctors neglected this essential area."

When I see them for the first time, some of these patients have already begun to "waste away," having lost significant percentages of their body weight. Lots of them complain that in the weeks or months immediately prior to seeing me, they always felt weak and to that point their advances in recovery had been negligible.

What many of these people fail to realize is that in essence their bodies have stalled or begun moving far too slow in the middle of life's proverbial freeway. Many problems with diet and various physical complications occurred due to internal damage caused by cancer and by side effects from rigorous, dangerous and sometimes unnecessary treatments previously received elsewhere.

During my initial examination process, some patients begin answering queries that they often had not been asked before. How often do you eat? What foods have been a prominent part of your typical daily diet since you've had cancer? What were typical meals that you regularly enjoyed before becoming ill? Where did you purchase most of your food, and how was it prepared?

Detoxification Becomes Vital

Following this first examination and my initial diagnosis, many patients need to learn the essentials of detoxification. By this stage some of these individuals still have residues of poisons or drugs in their bodies from previous treatments elsewhere. Others had not yet been treated before seeing me, but during my initial examinations of these patients their livers, gallbladders and intestines still contained the toxins that contributed to their cancers.

While certain qualified patients learn some or all of the detoxification strategies mentioned earlier, including the potential use of olive oil mixed with lemon juice, most also discover the foods they need to avoid in order to enable other antioxidant-rich meals to detoxify the body.

Right off the bat, some patients become surprised upon learning of the initial need to avoid white sugars, sugar substitutes, pastries, and commercially produced candies. At least in the detoxification phase the potentially strong antioxidant power of chocolate should be avoided. (We'll have much more discussion later on the vital need to enjoy dark chocolate, starting after the detoxification phase ends.)

Careful to avoid white rice, amid detoxification patients should also avoid cereals that have been processed, a manufacturing phase that makes them flaked or puffed. The same goes for white breads and products made from white flour including certain snacks, crackers and macaroni.

In addition, some homeopaths striving to help patients

detoxify urge them to avoid French fries, corn chips, potato chips—especially because salt is a definite "no-no" amid any serious detoxification regimen. Also stay away from red meat, especially those that have been processed, salted, smoked or fried, or preserved with nitrates.

Besides patients who feel they're addicted to sugary foods, those having some of the most challenges avoiding potentially harmful carcinogenic meals during detoxification aren't necessarily happy when discovering the need to forego coffee for that period. Alcoholics predictably get squeamish when learning of the need to avoid their favorite sugar-packed libations.

Some dietitians and nutrition experts also urge avoiding dairy products amid the initial three weeks of detoxification, while also keeping non-fertile or dried eggs off your menu for the duration of this important treatment phase.

Although this food-avoidance task might sound daunting at first, the vast majority of patients eagerly follow my advice. People with cancer typically become motivated to embrace recommended lifestyle changes designed to enable them to regain good health.

Great Foods for Detoxification

Lots of patients express delight upon learning that a wide variety of diverse foods help detoxification, according to a wide variety of reports by medical professionals including homeopaths.

Unsalted nuts can become formidable allies for boosting or maintaining energy amid detoxification, especially pecans, walnuts and almonds. Packed with protein, this high-energy food can help the body maintain vital strength and vibrancy throughout the day. Other helpful snacks during detoxification can include a wide variety of seeds ranging from peach, apricot, plumb, apple, prune, pumpkin and sunflower. Adding to your benefits, most seeds are loaded with antioxidants.

Among other foods frequently mentioned by some nutrition experts as excellent sources for detoxification:

Vegetables: Along with baked potatoes and homemade soups, enjoy a wide variety of organically grown vegetables—but only if raw or lightly steamed.

Sweets: Rather than highly processed snacks packed with white sugar, take delight in various natural foods including date sugars, carob, raw honey, sorghum and pure maple syrup, or treats made with these healthful ingredients.

Meat: While careful to avoid red meats, enjoy light amounts of turkey, chicken or the white flesh of fish.

Fruits: Enjoy all types of fresh fruits but only when organically grown. Remember, all fruits are metabolized in the sugar cycle.

Breads: Until recently, due to the advent of "Wheat Belly" whole wheat breads had almost universally been recommended by a majority of natural-medicine practitioners. Although the potential healthfulness of such crops has now been brought into question, a wide variety of other breads remain possible for detoxification. Among the most popular are breads made from corn or soy, or from other whole grains—particularly whole, non-wheat grains freshly ground and sprouted.

Cereals: Although you'll still need to avoid processed products that are flaked or puffed, you can use those comprised of unprocessed crops like cornmeal, and brown or wild rice.

The huge variety of other detoxification foods includes: fertile eggs poached or boiled, but only if eaten sparingly; dairy products like raw certified milk, cottage cheese, and yogurt but only if it's unsweetened; an expansive variety of vegetable juices and fruit juices; a wide range of sprouts including buckwheat, soy, lentil and alfalfa; and a huge variety of natural oils as long as they're unsaturated and cold-pressed. Finally, besides filtered water that is not sold in plastic, other helpful detoxification drinks can include nut milk, soy- and sesame-based beverages.

As you can undoubtedly see from reviewing these detoxification foods, the range of choices is wide enough to offer sufficient variety to keep the overall menu from seeming dull. Even so, if you're a cancer patient or a person assisting such an individual, adhering to this regimen will take stick-to-itiveness. Such meals can easily become a habit within your lifestyle, especially when starting with a focused "can-do" attitude.

Chapter 21 Summary

During chemotherapy and radiation treatments, eating the ideal nutritious foods is essential to survival and maintaining ideal weight so that that the person has enough physical energy to recover. But some oncologists fail to mention this critical issue. Many cancer patients need dieting assistance and encouragement from relatives, friends or medical professionals. Besides excessive weight loss, the failure to regularly eat ideal foods during chemo can lead to fuzzy thinking, fatigue, weakened immunity and increased dangers of internal bleeding. Good food supplies the biological energy necessary to give the patient a fighting chance at recovery. Thus, cancer patients amid the critically ill phase of illness need to remember that hope for recovery often hinges on their determination to eat well. Many of the best foods during this phase assist in detoxifying the body of harmful substances or drugs that some doctors use as treatments. Foods often mentioned as great for detoxification include fruits, unprocessed cereals, bread— particularly varieties without wheat; vegetables, sweet foods that lack white sugars like carob and raw honey, and light amounts of turkey, chicken the flesh of fish.

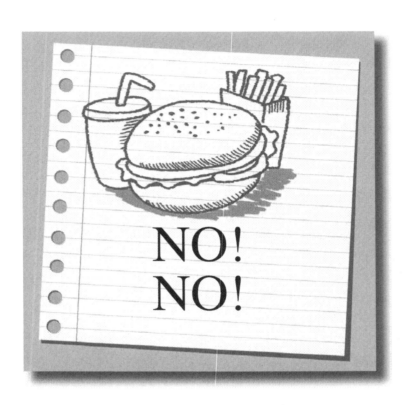

Chapter 22

Basic Strategies to Prevent Cancer

For patients and consumers who have never had cancer, we also list a wide range of diet-related recommendations on actions to take, and activities or foods to avoid as prevention measures. Of course, no one can ever guarantee that you'll never have cancer. Yet based on their experience and research, practitioners of natural health treatments have complied many diet-oriented recommendations on things "to do" and to "avoid doing" to minimize the risks of cancer. Among the most frequent diet-based suggestions:

Foods and Cooking Methods to Avoid

Soft drinks: Never drink these, even sugar-free brands. These harm or exhaust your adrenal glands and pancreas, integral to moving vital cancer-fighting hormones into the body and also transporting digestive enzymes that help absorb essential nutrients.

Processed foods: Avoid all processed foods, TV dinners, cookies, crackers, white breads or foods packed with sugar.

Coffee: Avoid drinking coffee, and if you do drink this, limit consumption to two cups daily.

Additives: Never eat foods containing additives, particularly chemicals used to preserve the meals.

Processed: Avoid processed milk that has been canned, dried, or homogenized.

Bad snacks: Steer clear of "foodless" snacks. Eat only whole, unprocessed foods without preservatives. Sugar-filled candy bars are a key example of foods to avoid.

Frying: Avoid fried foods, especially meals that are deep-fat fried such as chicken. Instead, choose roasted food. Chicken cooked this way is generally okay.

Commercial meat: Never buy commercial meats from animals that have eaten the non-steroidal estrogen "stilboestrol," or the meat of animals treated inhumanely.

Oils: Eating or cooking foods laden with hydrogenated shortenings or treated oils packed with preservatives could open a doorway to potential cancers.

Muscle meats: These portions of animals are sometimes considered less nutritious and potentially dangerous when eaten. Generally, the non-muscle portions of farm animals are considered more nutritious.

Breads: Avoid commercially produced white bread or foods that contain white breads, partly because these usually contain potentially harmful additives and preservatives.

Production process: Many scientists believe you're endangering your health, increasing the risks of cancer, when eating waxed, sprayed, dyed or fumigated vegetables and fruits.

Packaging: Vegetables and fruits offered in cans are often laden with harmful preservatives, overly sweetened with dangerous sugars, or overcooked so much that the food gets robbed of essential nutrients.

Eggs: Some studies indicate that cancer risks increase

when eating eggs from chickens that were force-fed, fattened by chemical-laden foods and living in small cages.

Foods to Eat and Cooking Methods to Use

Investigate: Become a "label detective" by checking packages for ingredients such as dangerous preservatives, high sugar content or elevated sodium levels.

Natural: Whenever possible, buy only natural or "raw" foods that have never been processed or filled with preservatives.

Dairy: Only drink certified raw milk whenever available.

Water: Make sure your water is distilled or filtered, possibly at home via your own mechanisms, and avoid buying water sold in plastic containers. Consumers who buy water or who filter their own water should also strive to ensure that they or their children receive adequate amounts of fluoride from sources other than public utilities.

Spoilage: Only buy foods that would spoil, and eat them before that process starts.

Produce: Make your yogurt, cottage cheese and ice cream at home, rather than buying processed and commercially produced food products that often are invariably laden with excessive sugars and preservatives.

Meats: Rather than always consuming one single area of animals such as ribs, use a variety of cuts, including the liver, heart and kidneys, or shortbreads and giblets.

Naturally raised: Buy only meats or fish that have been raised naturally in "free-roaming" environments, rather than those that lived in cages or within confined environments crammed with lots of similar animals.

Preserving: Buy good, fresh produce during the seasons that they're offered, sometimes freezing such foods for use later.

Frying: Use safflower oil, flaxseed oil or sesame oil, which have the highest smoke point.

Baking: When baking, for shortening use peanut oil, sesame oil, soy or safflower oil made with no preservatives in a cold process.

Growth: People unable to or unwilling to grow their own fruits and vegetables should purchase these foods only if they have been grown organically.

Eggs: Avoid non-fertile eggs, buying only fertile eggs because they're less likely to contain sprays or antibiotics.

Chapter 22 Summary

In preventing or treating cancer, homeopaths and dietitians have a lengthy list of recommendations of foods and cooking methods to either avoid or to use.

Chapter 23

Control Inflammation Complications

Inflammation suffered on a chronic, continuous and debilitating level often afflicts cancer patients due to their disease or complications arising from treatment. The challenge for many health professionals and their patients becomes finding and using effective natural foods capable of eliminating or alleviating this condition.

Unlike when a person sprains an ankle or breaks a bone, inflammation suffered by cancer patients often emerges internally in the bones, soft tissues and solid organs.

To get a clear understanding of this, keep in mind that rather than being the "actual, primary injury," inflammation serves as the body's natural response to adverse events such as invading free radicals. In fact, on a regular basis your body and the bodies of the people around you are continually producing various levels of biological inflammation fighters. This is done in reaction to everything from chemicals, invading organisms, germs, allergies and other threats.

Inflammation is a typical and normal reaction to such bodily invaders or injuries. Specifically, swelling often occurs when your body generates extra protective white blood cells, pushing these valuable allies into the bloodstream. When swelling occurs on the body's surface, the symptoms are seen or felt as pain, aching, ulcerations, and the appearance of swelling on bodily surface areas along with a reddish color and a slight sense of heat. Internally, this occurs when your white blood cells help with the installation of new healthy cells to replace damaged tissue.

For cancer patients, this challenge can emerge as potentially formidable, especially when interfering with: the body's ability to effectively absorb nutrients; and the effectiveness of medications or various treatments. Another significant factor hinges on the essential healthy interaction between the body's various organs that are necessary for resuming and maintaining good health.

When Inflammation Goes off Kilter
Under ideal conditions, the human body uses a variety of interactions with inflammation to heal injuries or to battle invaders. Yes, swelling, clotting and even some fevers can actually be "good" for generating your short- and long-term recovery from a variety of injuries and ailments. These recoveries are all made possible by the phenomenon of inflammation.

The critical importance of finding and ingesting natural foods to help control inflammation becomes especially important when we consider various complications that might arise. Although the body's natural inflammation process typically "works miracles," the same systems sometimes generate enzymes that play a significant part in generating new blood vessels—even within the bodies of mature adults. Under healthy conditions, this development might enable the body to send more nutrients and white blood cells to the injurious area.

Yet as if invading aliens from another planet, tumors—some

of them initially too small to easily detect—essentially "hijack" these new blood vessels. With the devilishness of pirates, the tumors then essentially rob oxygen and nutrients from the very new blood vessels that the body had created as a protective or healing mechanism.

This interactive process essentially "feeds upon itself," with the growing tumors and the body's natural inflammation processes steadily promoting each other. As cancer worsens, spreads and strengthens, the body naturally creates invader-fighting white blood cells that the diseases eventually uses to thrive even more—getting closer to the goal of the death of itself, and the potential demise of the patient as well. Along the way as the patient's overall condition steadily worsens, the pirate-like cancer within its own realm becomes "healthy" and "vibrant" in steadily increasing amounts. Such conditions, of course, are unhealthy for the patient, especially when cancer moves or metastasizes from its original site to other organs or regions of the body.

What Foods Cause Inflammation?

Through numerous studies, researchers have pinpointed foods suspected as possible causes of the types of internal inflammations that are deemed most likely to lead to cancer.

Not surprisingly, scientists blame meals loaded with trans fats and food packed with white sugar as primary culprits. Another important discovery indicated that certain types of oil are less prone to lead to such potentially harmful conditions.

All this becomes increasingly interesting when also accounting for the fact that the very processes of "being alive" as a mammal naturally creates potentially cancer-causing free radicals within humans. You see, the body mixes oxygen that you breathe with nutrients. This "oxidation" process creates the energy needed by the body to sustain itself and remain alive. However, naturally creating potential dangers for itself, this same essential process pulls a single electron from all molecules or atoms as they combine with oxygen. This creates dangerous free radicals.

Even among healthy people without cancer the body is essentially loaded with "robbers" that steal non-stop, and "cops" that strive to throw them into the biological slammer. Far more serious than a goofy "cops and robbers" film, within your body molecules are continually losing electrons. Following the dictates of Mother Nature, each unattached electron strives to "pair up" with another loose electron; within nature, electrons invariably come in pairs.

The "stealing" continues unabated, even in healthy people by efficiently generating the energy they need to live. However, this process hailed as the "metabolism" sometimes gets seriously hampered by the foods a person eats or by other invaders. Sadly, toxic food sometimes unsettles the normally healthy "cops and robber" process, which also sometimes gets hampered by heavy metals and a wide variety of other negative lifestyle factors such as smoking or when people allow ourselves to become obese.

Toxins Create an Imbalance

With everything leading to the possibility of cancer-causing inflammation, excessive amounts of toxins often generate an imbalance within the body's ability to process and absorb essential nutrients. When pushed to excessive levels, the result is oxidative stress that pushes the proverbial "cops and robbers" into overdrive.

Unless the body successfully manages this process, the oxidation system spins out of control as if the equivalent of thousands of murderers who have simultaneously escaped from prison. The white blood cells, particularly killer T-cells, do their best to nab these culprits amid the equivalent of a community-wide riot. Yet even if the white blood cells have a fairly high degree of success during the initial chaos, the body's natural protective mechanisms have invariably created inflammation.

With planning, specific care and lifestyle adjustments, people with cancer and consumers everywhere can essentially minimize or lessen the probability of such calamity. Eating meals loaded with antioxidants can go a long way toward preventing the body from suffering from oxidative stress or excess inflammation.

Avoid Becoming Obese

As stated earlier, having a fat belly significantly increases your probability of getting cancer. Being overweight accelerates or sparks oxidative stress. Danger levels increase when taking into account the undeniable fact that excessive body weight also often leads to potentially deadly diabetes, heart disease, strokes and other serious ailments.

Some patients ask how "being fat" can result in cancer.

This flab, often called "visceral fat," serves as a primary place for your body to store excess energy that usually results from eating too many calories, ingesting the wrong foods, or when failing to exercise enough to burn these excess calories. The fat deposits also store toxins in the body.

The potential danger of visceral fat intensifies when considering the fact that it's far different from intramuscular fat interspersed throughout the body's skeletal muscles, and even subcutaneous fat under your skin.

Unlike the excess energy that's stored elsewhere in the body, sometimes used for protecting muscles or organs, visceral fat occasionally sends out excessive levels of what doctors call "cytokine" cells. In terms that lay people can easily understand, these are signaling molecules that transmit information among the body's cellular structures. Technically, this is the body's miraculous "intracellular communication" switchboard. Essentially, your cells are telling each other, "send more of this here, and send less of that there," or "the body needs to generate more of a certain enzyme in order to handle a particular problem."

Yet when communicating their own needs, due to their over-abundance within the body, visceral fats might sometimes inadvertently force usually helpful white blood cells to "misfire"—thereby creating potentially harmful excess inflammation.

The possibility for danger occasionally becomes even worse because, in the view of some scientists, the body's natural insulin sometimes plays a role in producing inflammation. The critical factor here emerges from the unchangeable fact that insulin, produced within the pancreas, regulates how the cells of fat tissues absorb and use glucose that the body transports via the blood. As a necessary energy source for maintaining life glucose plays an essential role for digestion. When that process receives incorrect or excessive intracellular signals, scientists believe, the body's ability to process toxins and to regulate free radicals sometimes gets hampered—eventually resulting in cancer.

Check for Warning Signs

As you modify your diet or exercise in an effort to maintain a flat belly or to lose stomach fat, you'll need to consume primarily antioxidant foods and possibly decrease your average daily caloric intake. Amid this phase, although never attempting to diagnose your condition—something only a physician should do, you should check for potential warning signs that your body might have excessive internal inflammation. Among possible signals:

Breathing: Is your nose continually stuffy for no obvious reason, at chronic or persistent levels without any known or apparent allergies?

Mouth: Are your gums puffy or overly red, even bleeding, although you regularly brush and floss your teeth every day and use mouthwash that's usually effective in removing or preventing plaque?

Joints: Are your joints continually sore without any other known underlying reason, perhaps even to the point of full-blown arthritis?

Other signals: Additional possible signs might sometimes seem less evident, but they should be considered when suffered continually or frequently—such as skin eruptions like eczema and acne far past the teen years, headaches and digestive difficulties.

Once you begin suspecting that your body might have excessive inflammation, only a doctor or certified medical professional can formally make such a diagnosis.

Are you Sensitive to Some Foods?

When suspecting that foods you eat might cause inflammation, some homeopaths and dietitians recommend specialized tests to determine if your body is sensitive to certain meals. Medical experts can sometimes determine this by conducting a food-sensitivity panel that helps determine if you're allergic to or have adverse reactions to everything from wheat to meat or of even dairy products like pasteurized milk.

When these tests identify a specific food as a suspected problem, eliminating those from the diet sometimes soon eliminates the adverse symptoms of possible inflammation. Once again, we have a prime example of the age-old adage "you are what you eat," in some instances the very foods that might cause cancer.

Upon learning these basics for the first time, many people become increasingly aware of the essential need to take a pro-active and continual role in helping to ensure continued good health, or to rebound from illnesses including cancer. Luckily, there are several other medical tests that also determine the probability of—or the actual observation of—excessive internal inflammation. Among these examinations:

Blood tests: This specialized health check identifies your body's level of what biologists call a "C-reactive protein." Found primarily within the blood, this specific protein increases within the blood as the body's specialized but automatic response to inflammation. The body uses C-reactive proteins as a natural, internally generated physiological system that interacts with the surfaces of cells that are already dead or dying. The body sharply increases its production of C-reactive protein, sometimes called "CRP," formed in the liver in order to respond to signals released by fat cells and by macrophages that assist in the body's immunity. Through many years as a physician while developing the Forsythe Anti-Cancer Diet, I have determined that taking a CRP blood test is an essential diagnostic tool for cancer patients or for individuals who might have the disease. When the test shows that a patient has excessive CRP levels, I immediately develop a treatment regimen and change to the person's diet. Thereafter, the individual needs to have a similar test at least every three months to determine the levels of progress, while also helping me to modify the individual's treatments if necessary. Also, rather than only concentrating on CRP, at the onset of diagnosis I also check for a variety of other potential inflammatory markers within the blood.

Thermography: Under the direction of a physician, certified and licensed medical professionals use infrared imaging devices—partly in order to detect levels of heat within tissue that contains cancer, or is suspected of having precancerous features like inflammation. Research indicates that the same inflammation factors considered as cancerous or precancerous always generate heat. Thus, scientists consider thermal imaging tests as exceptional ways to detect cancer or precancerous conditions, even in the very early formation stages in various areas of the body—particularly the breasts. These examination devices used by medical teams under the supervision of licensed thermologists enable physicians to review images captured by thermography cameras. From within the bodies of people with cancer or precancerous tissues, the devices can detect heat where early or advanced inflammation results as in interaction with an accelerated metabolism caused partly by the vibrant interactions of protective white blood cells.

Fibrinogen: Every person needs his or her blood to clot properly in order to maintain good health. Cancer patients clot easily. When responding to signals of inflammation anywhere within the body, the liver produces a specialized protein called "fibrinogen." This natural, internally generated substance immediately and specifically targets inflammation. For cancer patients with elevated fibrinogen, homeopaths sometimes recommend foods high in antioxidants and natural anti-coagulants to assist in bringing this substance to healthier levels—thereby increasing the efficiency of blood flow and preventing thrombosis.

Learn to Lower Your Inflammation

Besides a wide variety of medications designed to lower inflammation, people with excessive amounts of this condition should follow the instructions of their dietitians or homeopaths in modifying their ingestion of oils. Many scientists say that from among all possible foods, oils play perhaps the most significant role when interacting with various chemicals and biological

221

interactions that cause, minimize or decrease swelling.

In a sense, fats act as if pre-programmed mathematical configurations within an electronic calculator. Under normal operation, all equations are pre-set to occur in a certain reliable and predictable way. But when an unhealthy or ill-advised fat is digested that substance can essentially trick your body's normally efficient processes from reaching the correct conclusions on how and when to generate certain essential chemicals and enzymes. "Bad oil" can cause your body's entire natural internal computer to collapse, ultimately forcing biological mechanisms to reach the "wrong" conclusions—thereby internally producing natural chemicals and enzymes that emerge as ineffective at reducing inflammation.

This, in turn, can subsequently lead the body to produce even more inefficient substances, since the initial tabulations of your internal chemistry were "wrong." Think of it this way. When calculating your total annual income by adding up your monthly revenues, the ultimate sum will be wrong if you initially input incorrect information for the months of January, February and March.

On a biological level, internal calculations misfire due to eating inadequate or unhealthy oils, generating a host of potentially destructive situations. Within cells, the damage occurs primarily when "bad oils" disrupt or adversely change a necessary layer of lipid fat within every cell. In healthy people, lipid fats allow waste to exit a cell, while also enabling vital nutrients to enter the same biological structure. Yet health complications gradually or suddenly emerge when "bad" fats block or clog up cell membranes, preventing or curtailing the proper entering and exiting of nutrients and waste.

James W. Forsythe, M.D., H.M.D.

Trans Fats Pose Extreme Danger

By far, the most dangerous unhealthy food within this sector are trans fats, found nowhere in nature except within a limited amounts of fat and milk from cattle and sheep—but prevalent in grocery stores, restaurants and fast-food joints. A decrease in the need for refrigeration and increases in shelf life are among primary factors why some food manufacturers and distributors use trans fats.

Understandably, then, healthy people and people with cancer should refrain from buying any food product containing trans fats or from ordering restaurant meals having them. To do otherwise, I tell patients, is "to literally invite the Grim Reaper to play devilish games within your body."

Sometimes called "unsaturated fats," foods within the trans fat category contain double-carbon bonding within their molecular structures. These unique atomic-level bonding structures wreak havoc on the natural process of supplying the human body's cells with critical nutrients.

The unique and destructive chemical characteristics of trans fats are created when manufacturers or cooks generate polyunsaturated fats during the production process.

Besides opening up the biological doorway to potential cancer, trans fats also increase the levels of unhealthy LDL cholesterol—thereby sharply increasing the development of potentially fatal coronary heart disease.

Studies vary sharply on the potential dangers of certain types of trans fats. According to some news articles, research conducted in Canada indicated that trans fats generated from beef and dairy products might be beneficial. While laboratory results vary on this issue, depending on which specific studies are involved, overall from the view of many homeopaths this would indicate that trans

223

fats from hydrogenated vegetable shortening are far worse than those naturally produced within animals.

However, a wide variety of other studies indicate that all forms of trans fats are equally unhealthful—no matter where they come from.

"You need to avoid all trans fats, no matter how they're made," I tell patients. "The possible dangers are just too great for you to risk your health."

Hidden Biological Problems Revealed

On a cellular level, the carbon atoms of unsaturated fat contain at least one—and possibly more—double bonds. As a result, the molecular structure contains fewer bonds attached to hydrogen and thereby these fats have fewer atoms of that element.

Although many homeopaths proclaim otherwise, based on various news stories and medical articles some researchers believe there is no link between trans fats and cancer. In fact, even the American Cancer Society has proclaimed that any relationship "has not been determined" between cancer and trans fats.

To the contrary, however, at least one study at Oxford did indeed find what its researchers concluded that there is a direct correlation between trans fats and prostate cancer.

Adding to my concern, additional research conducted in France showed that people who ate high levels of trans fats may increase by 75 percent their risk of breast cancer. Additional research concluded that eating trans fats might increase belly fat and rise overall body weight, precursors for potential cancer.

Consumers Take Decisive Action

Highly concerned and in some cases enraged by the detrimental effects of trans fats, consumers worldwide have taken varying levels of action to eliminate or to curtail the sale and consumption of such food. Among the many other potential health problems often cited, some of them disputed by varying studies, are Alzheimer's Disease, type 2 diabetes, liver dysfunction, mental depression and infertility within women.

Until 2006, U.S. consumers rarely knew the levels of trans fats in specific types and brands of foods that they bought. That changed when food manufacturers were required to start labeling trans fat levels on food packaging, as required by regulations enacted in 2003 by the U.S. Food and Drug Administration (FDA.)

Despite this potentially positive development, according to some published reports the FDA has indicated that every day the average American eats a whopping 2.6 grams of trans fats. If true, this means that the a typical person in the United States eats a combined 949 grams of trans fats yearly, or from my perspective "more than two pounds of pure cancer-causing, heart-damaging poisons." I suspect that this over-consumption of this extremely dangerous food occurs due to six primary reasons.

Knowledge: Many consumers simply do not know what's in the foods that they eat, and a percentage of the population lacks any concept of the dangers imposed by trans fat.

Confusion: Even among those aware of this issue, some food buyers may become confused by the wording on food labels. For instance, consumers might become confused or "tricked" by large-letter labels that say things like "low trans fats," when in fact the FDA specifically has not yet set the definition of what such terms mean. Thus, packing that largely claims the food is low in trans fats could actually contain dangerously high levels of that substance. When this happens, the listed levels are set at arbitrarily amounts designated by, or essentially "picked out of the sky" by manufacturers.

Restaurants: When eating at restaurants diners typically have no way of knowing whether specific meals contain trans fats, unless these consumers ask specific questions

Parties and families: People at parties or social gatherings typically lack the specific, in-depth knowledge about what is being served. And, many family members typically are "at the mercy" of relatives, relying on whatever meals are bought or prepared for them.

Institutions: The administrators and managers of major institutions including elementary school cafeterias and even hospitals might lack definable guidelines from the labeling on packages of food amassed for large institutions.

Inadequate levels: Heightening the public's overall level of concern, come consumers strongly complain that FDA rules allow producers and distributors to list a food as free of trans fat if the product contains no more than 0.5 grams per serving. I'm among those who worry that this arbitrary, pre-set ruling might emerge as extremely detrimental to the predominant health of American society.

"Overall, big companies and our government are toying with the public's health," I tell patients. "Unless you take a pro-active role within this arena, you might end up eating way too many trans fats—hindering your cancer-recovery efforts, or increasing the probability that you will eventually suffer from the disease."

Although various state and local governments nationwide have taken separate, unrelated efforts to ban or limit trans fats, much more needs to be done to protect the public health. At present, the decisions that you make will emerge as the most important factor in generating your personal outcome—good or bad.

Manufacturers Responded Positively

Although the manufacture and distribution of trans fats remains pervasive, to their credit at least some major multi-billion-dollar companies have taken positive steps to reverse the situation. For instance, the manufacturer of Crisco—a partially hydrogenated vegetable shortening—the J.M. Smucker Company—began cutting soybean oil with the solid saturated palm oil in 2004 when developing a new formulation.

A handful of other food makers also eliminated or reduced trans fat. In 2004, the flagship Becel™ brand of the Uniliver corporation cut trans fat from margarine sold in Canada. At least one major Southeast Asia company that produces confectionary fats and trans fat-free baked goods for huge U.S. corporations started making margarine that researchers deemed less harmful.

Some companies voluntarily made similar reductions, while numerous corporations faced lawsuits from consumer organizations to stop using trans fat. Among notable cases:

Craft Foods: Settled a 2003 lawsuit filed by Ban Trans Fat Com Inc., agreeing that in the production of Oreo™ cookies it would find trans fat substitutes.

Arby's: In 2007, reduced trans fat in various foods, eliminating it from French fries.

Kentucky Fried Chicken: Often called "KFC," at its U.S. restaurants, in 2007 the company started using a zero trans fat soy bean oil to make its original recipe, replacing partially hydrogenated soybean oil. The company started using various other substitutes outside the United States.

Taco Bell: Removed trans fat, or starting offering foods free of the substance, impacting 15 separate meals.

McDonald's: Following years of delay and testing,

announced in 2007 that trans fats were being phased out of its fries.

Other companies taking action included: Disney, which removed trans fat from its theme park meals in late 2007; and the Girl Scouts of the USA, which reduced trans fat in its cookies in 2006, to less than 0.5 grams per serving.

Always Remain Vigilant

Despite the strides made by consumers and corporations, people worldwide need to remain vigilant in efforts to avoid trans fat. Although some researchers might tell the public otherwise, I'm among doctors who insist that this dangerous substance is likely a major contributor to at least some cancers—especially of the breast and of the prostate. Among my top recommendations:

Restaurants: When ordering in restaurants, always ask specifically if a meal or food item has no trans fat or less than 0.5 grams of it per serving. If the food server is unable to give a definitive answer, order another item or go to a different dining facility.

Packaging: If packaging says "low trans fat" or "no trans fat," but lists less than 0.5 grams of it per serving on the more detailed label, buy a different product.

Activist: As a consumer, as a parent, as a family member or as a concerned citizen, take decisive action to eliminate trans fat from school lunch menus and from college cafeterias.

Youngsters: Prohibit your children from buying snacks like certain French fries or packaged muffin treats containing trans fat.

By remaining vigilant on this critical issue, you can likely increase your own life span, prevent unnecessary weight gain, and protect the health of your relatives.

Chapter 23 Summary

Internal inflammation is often deemed a major cause of cancer, even when the internal swelling occurs naturally. Inflammation usually occurs when the body sends extra protective white blood cells to a particular bodily region that is attacked by invaders that may include carcinogens. This swelling exacerbates the problem, generating new blood vessels that feeds tumors and enables the disease to thrive. Foods high in free radicals and certain unhealthy oils are sometimes blamed for creating these cancer-causing conditions. Obese people with excessive visceral fat sometimes suffer internal inflammation that leads to cancer. Everyone, especially heavy individuals, should check for warning signs of possible internal inflammation. Possible warning signs include chronically stuffy noses, bleeding gums, aching joints, and persistent skin problems. Sensitivity to certain foods also can generate internal inflammation. Doctors can perform various tests to look for signs of such conditions. A primary dietary strategy for avoiding inflammation is to avoid eating trans fat, also called "unsaturated fats," often blamed for generating free radicals that cause inflammation. Always check food labels, and avoid foods that contain trans fats or listed as having low amounts of that substance.

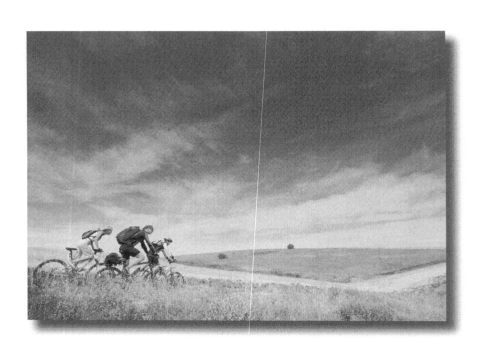

Chapter 24

Minimize
Your Inflammation Risks

While eliminating trans fat remains an essential strategy in minimizing potential inflammation, you should continually employ other lifestyle habits deemed effective in achieving this vital goal. Among the most essential:

Rotate foods: Continually change the foods and meals that you eat the most often during periods of several weeks. Some dietitians and homeopaths believe this strategy enables people to avoid overloading their bodies with foods likely to generate sensitive symptoms or that would generate allergic reactions. Sometimes the body lacks enough energy to effectively process specific foods, with these propensities varying with each individual's DNA or the damage caused by toxins. Rotating foods also might allow you to determine what foods, if any, are the likely causes of your adverse reactions. Just as important, from my view temporarily eliminating certain foods from your diet might give your immunity system adequate time to naturally re-energize.

Exercise: Especially when done in moderation, exercise obviously can emerge as an essential strategy in any weight-loss diet program. Some studies also show that exercising several times monthly at the very minimum can help lessen the probability that various tumors might develop, including breast cancer. All along, however, at least from the view of some researchers, the "overtraining syndrome" can generate intracellular communication that causes internal inflammation. Even so, in the long run exercise may strengthen the immune system against various potential ailments including cancer. I urge everyone, particularly patients who exercise, to get adequate sleep and rest to enable the body to heal from the potential negative side effects of physical activity. My popular book first published in 2009, "The Healing Power of Sleep," gives essential advice on how to get adequate rest. Another effective tactic also becomes exercising in moderation. Rather than running at a break-neck pace or jogging non-stop for hours, consider walking steadily for less than 45 minutes at a stretch—no matter what your age.

Antioxidants: At this juncture, the earlier discussion of the ongoing need to eat antioxidants should be increasingly apparent. When taken at continually high levels, these vital qualities can fortify the body's ability to prevent free radicals from generating inflammation or causing oxidative stress.

White sugars: The excessive intake of white sugar can catapult intermittent pulses of high-level insulin, raising blood sugar levels—often deemed a significant factor in triggering the body's inflammation processes. In scientific terms, this means that you should strive to decrease your body's "glycemic load."

Omega-3 fats: Various studies consistently conclude that the average American eats far too many potentially harmful omega-6 fats, and not enough healthy omega-3 fats. Researchers believe that omega-6 fatty acids, often from foods like grains and nuts, ignite the body's inflammation processes. Conversely, omega-3 fatty acids, often found in sardines, and halibut, can sharply decrease any propensity toward inflammation. Besides from supplements, the many other potential sources of omega-3 include walnuts, flaxseeds, pumpkin seeds and leafy vegetables. Although omega-6 can spark inflammation, doctors insist that this substance and also omega-3 fall within the distinct category of "essential fatty acids." This means that people need to eat and efficiently absorb both of them in order to enjoy good health. Mammals including humans lack the ability to internally produce these specific and necessary fats, and therefore must ingest them. Thus, people undergoing so-called "fat-free" diets need to remain cautious, mindful of these essential needs. In fact, the body's natural need for these fats is so critical that eating omega-3 contained within specific varieties of fish often proves effective in reversing mental depression. Some researchers also believe that the body absorbs omega-3 far more efficiently from fish than from plants. The body must undergo more complex metabolic work to process omega3-from plants, while humans easily absorb the same substance when derived from fish, scientists say. Some fish species have far more beneficial omega-3 than others. White fish like cod, flatfish and haddock only have oil in their livers, most living close to the seafloor. The fillet fish containing the most abundant omega-3 prefer living near the surface, including sardines, and herring—plus much larger varieties like trout, salmon and mackerel. Besides lessening the possibility of inflammation that could lead to cancer, people who eat oily fish also lessen their chances of suffering from a variety of other ailments including Alzheimer's or the steady progression of age-related macular degeneration. While also hailed as helpful to cardiovascular health, oily fish should be eaten at least two times weekly, according to several medical reports from the United Kingdom. Despite these many positive attributes, some officials including the U.S.

Environmental Protection Agency recommend limiting oily fish in order to minimize the dangers of eating animals exposed to methyl-mercury. According to a 2004 report by the Scientific Advisory Commission on Nutrition, the recommended EPA restrictions apply to certain oily fish—shark, swordfish and marlin, and tuna to a lesser extent. The reported maximum exposure level is 0.1 micrograms daily for every kilogram of body weight. Based on the various reports I've seen, researchers seem to strongly recommend having at least two servings of 4.9 ounces of oily fish weekly, but no more than four servings. While omega-3 coming primarily from fish oil is deemed extremely healthy for us and necessary for optimal health, the potential dangers of mercury poisoning from such animals is often critical. These conflicting factors emerge as a considerable oxymoron. Mercury poisoning can be extremely toxic to the body, particularly the lungs, brain and kidney. Adverse symptoms can include severely impaired vision, speech and coordination. Luckily, for people worried about the dangers of eating oily fish, scientists say that the level of severity from mercury poisoning hinges largely on the duration and amounts of exposure. Thus, at least if researchers are to be believed, anyone who eats no more than four servings of oily fish each week should have very little fear of mercury contamination.

Chapter 24 Summary

To minimize risks of internal inflammation, people need to exercise, limit their daily calorie intake, rotate foods, eat lots of antioxidants, avoid white sugars and eat plenty of omega-3 fats often found in sardines, halibut and other oily fish. Some fish have far more omega-3 content than others; generally, you should seek fish species that live mostly far below the surface. Omega-3 fats are essential to good health, lessening the probability of Alzheimer's disease and certain age-related muscle degeneration diseases. You should limit servings to no more than four servings of oily fish weekly in order to avoid excessive, harmful consumption of methyl-mercury.

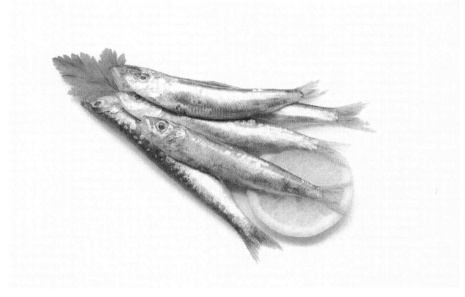

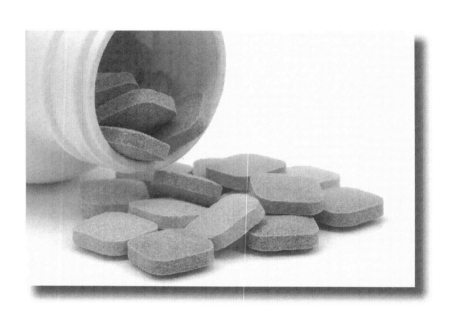

Chapter 25

Dietary Supplements

The use of dietary supplements can serve as a formidable tool within the Forsythe Anti-Cancer Diet regimen, particularly for patients who need to quickly fortify their bodies with essential vitamins and nutrients.

Usually taken orally via capsules, as an overall category supplements are deemed as potentially beneficial. In fact, an international book on accepted standards—the "Codex Alimentarius"—includes these substances as a category of food.

For the vast majority of cases where cancer patients see only standard oncologists, the possibility of using supplements as an integral part of treatment is never mentioned. This blatant, intentional oversight angers some homeopaths.

You see, doctors have a responsibility to give their cancer patients a "fighting chance," even when a cancer patient reaches the critical stage IV. Particularly among patients who have dropped huge percentages of body weight and lost strength, supplements can enable them to ingest the elements they need to recover. In fact, from my view the potential use of supplements is so critical that any oncologist who fails to offer them is flat-out performing a disservice to the very patients that they're sworn to treat. Among the primary potential benefits from nutrient-packed supplements:

Vitamins: Often critical in enabling cells to have a "fighting chance" at battling cancer, minimizing impacts of the disease, or in preventing it from spreading.

Minerals: This involves the critical and necessary delivery of substances like zinc, magnesium and iron to fortify the body's continual war against disease and infection.

Fatty acids: These substances, especially fish oil, can help the body minimize the potential impact of symptoms such as inflammation that when left untreated can lead to cancer or promote the spread of the disease.

Detoxify: Some supplements help the body remove toxins that stall or block the cancer recovery process. Under specific situations, detoxification also can sometimes assist overweight people whose bodies are "starved for food" because toxic overload prevents their digestive systems from absorbing essential nutrients.

Weakness: For patients who have become extremely weak due to cancer and from treatments including chemo, an adequate and well-timed supplement regimen can enable them to steadily gain strength—opening a potential pathway for recovery.

Engage Professionals

You should view with suspicion anyone who boldly claims that a particular supplement "will cure cancer" or prevent the disease. Never seriously consider or purchase supplements from a person or company that makes such rosy pitches.

Instead, you should only receive and use dietary supplements under the recommendation of a medical professional. Best-case situations involve homeopaths or dietitians who select supplements designed for your specific needs.

All along, patients and consumers everywhere should remain mindful of potentially false claims. In October 2012, the U.S. Department of Health and Human Services (DHSS) announced results of its research into the accuracy of labeling on dietary supplements.

According to several news reports, of the 127 immune-boosting and weight-loss supplements studied by DHSS, a whopping 20 percent had labeling that made false claims such as curing diseases.

Some of these bogus and potentially fraudulent labels even claimed cures for cancer, AIDS or diabetes, the agency's investigators reported. Shocked by these findings, many health industry analysts became concerned that some patients might end up making the ill-advised decision of stopping their prescription medications, or avoiding medical professionals. This, in turn, could lead to disastrous results among patients who rely on bogus claims and ineffective products.

Seek a Balanced Approach

Despite the occasional media firestorms on this issue, patients need to remain aware that supplements can emerge as important cancer-fighting tools when correctly administered. As a medical professional, I would never even entertain the idea of proclaiming any particular supplement as a "be-all, and end-all" cancer cure.

Be that as it may, however, the media performs a serious disservice to the public by recklessly proclaiming or implying that all supplements are dangerous—and that patients should use only prescription drugs. To the contrary, now in my fifth decade as a physician, I can proclaim beyond any reasonable doubt whatsoever that many of the expensive drugs that our federal agencies tout are worthless or even extremely harmful to patients.

Herein emerges a primary reason why I have a professional responsibility to give my clinic's patients referrals to appropriate types of supplements. This is done only based on my chemo-sensitivity reports and my staff's professional diagnosis of specific aspects of a patient's condition.

On the flip side of this proverbial coin, our nation's huge federal agencies that are supposed to be protecting the public put consumers in extreme jeopardy everywhere. How dare "the feds" strive to dissuade the public from using natural remedies such as Vitamin C, while steering patients to poisons like chemotherapy? What right does the almighty government have to dictate your health care, and to decide what potential treatments you should avoid?

Well, from my view—similar to that of many homeopaths, everything comes down to the "almighty dollar," coupled with a corrupt government that is weighted toward Big Pharma and Big Food. Remember, armies of lobbyists for those industries swarm through the halls of Congress, bullying our politicians while also playing a devilish role in why and how large federal agencies ban certain natural treatments or strive to convince the public not to use them. Foolish and lazy, the mainstream news media sometimes unwittingly or recklessly serves an integral role in helping to pull off this charade.

Become Vigilant

Refusing to get hoodwinked into believing all of the government's hogwash, cancer patients need to take a pro-active role on this issue. With recovery as the ultimate goal, if you have the disease or you're related to such a person, take a vigilant role in aggressively seeking definitive, honest answers. Among them:

Availability: Ask your doctor or medical professional why the possibility of supplements has never been mentioned. With similar intensity, inquire about why a dietitian has never been recommended.

Referrals: If the physician balks at your initial questions, ask if that person can refer you to a medical professional capable of considering supplements as among your viable, potentially effective treatment options.

Costs: Inquire about costs, since expenses are an issue for most patients. Why, for instance, would you need to spend lots of money on an expensive drug, when a natural, fairly inexpensive supplement might generate similar or even better benefits?

Experience: Ask your medical professional how much experience he or she has in recommending supplements? If this person has never recommended supplements, or universally advises against using them, at least in my view you should seriously consider finding another doctor or dietitian.

Claims: Does the recommended supplement make a 100-percent claim that it cures or alleviates cancer in all instances? Remember, if and when you ever hear such pitches, take such acclimations as "lies" and immediately go elsewhere.

Safety: With just as much urgency, you'll need to ask about the safety and potential dangers of specific high-cost drugs and of certain supplements. Which product is safest, with less potentially negative side effects? Intermixed with these criteria, which product is likely to get the best results? Also, can certain supplements and drugs be used simultaneously, and—if so—what are potential unique side effects from using them together?

History: When using specific supplements, what results have been experienced by the doctor's typical patients with similar medical conditions in the past? Would these average outcomes likely generate health improvements for you? If so, what, if anything, should prevent you from being provided with or recommended to similar natural remedies?

Prescription Issues

Within the United States, other potential issues can stem from the fact that many specific brands of supplements do not require a prescription. Thus, many formulations of such products are readily available within the open marketplace, including at many grocery stories, pharmacies and giant store chains like Wal-Mart.

But when buying at such retailers, are you qualified to make such critical health decisions? For most consumers who lack integral medical knowledge, how can those individuals know what supplements might work best for their specific conditions?

Also, there might be a danger that consumers wanting to seek out "cures" or "remedies" on their own without the benefit of professional advice might be setting themselves up for long-term heartache. The specific concern here stems from the fact that self-diagnosis and self-treatments would prevent the person from getting a thorough professional medical evaluation and diagnosis.

By ignoring doctors and refusing to see them altogether, a person might develop serious stage IV cancers that go undetected until the potential end-of-life clock starts ticking. Through the years, I cannot even begin to estimate the number of patients that I've helped, who waited far too long to get professional medical help.

Certainly, any total reliance on potential remedies without professional assistance can evolve into a "fool's game," where the patient becomes the potential loser. The same goes for people assisting their children or other relatives. As a caring family member, you want to give your loved ones the best chances possible of being diagnosed early, and getting the best treatment under the care of a qualified professional.

In addition, any person who already knows that he or she has cancer and then tries to "play doctor" by seeking out and using his own supposed cures such as dietary supplements very likely sets himself up for failure. With all these critical factors clearly understood, avoid getting into a position where you might have to say on your deathbed, "One of my biggest regrets is that I insisted on acting like a doctor myself. If only I had bothered to see one..."

Get a Second Chance at Life

Although dietary supplements should never be used as the only treatment method, even while under a doctor's care, from my experience they can go a long way toward helping in a cancer patient's overall recovery.

Fully cognizant of this fact, consumers also need to understand that supplements are in a different class from typical major-brand multi-vitamins found at most pharmacies and grocery stores. Based on a wide spectrum of medical research, coupled with professional experiences during the early stages of my career, I'm among physicians who acknowledge that standard multi-vitamins do little or nothing to generate good health.

All along, a limited number of studies have indicated that using multi-vitamins can spark at least some positive results. For instance, as reported by ABC News in October 2012, a comprehensive study of 15,000 men suggested that taking multi-vitamins daily might slightly lower their cancer risks. In this study published in the "Journal of the American Medical Association," half the men received multi-vitamins and the others got placebos over an 11-year study period—with average ages at about 65. The study's lead author, Harvard Medical School professor Michael

Gaziano, was quoted as saying, "Our study shows a modest but significant benefit in cancer prevention." The study used a multi-vitamin designed to reverse vitamin deficiencies.

Despite such positive findings, the vast majority of vitamins and mineral elements from such pills slide through the body without being absorbed, ending up in the sewer systems. The human body has difficulty or even an inability to process multi-vitamins, which usually are not delivered into the digestive tract in a natural, easily absorbed form.

By contrast, at least from what I've seen, the vast majority of dietary supplements come in capsules that are easily absorbed—usually natural, leafy substances rather than encapsulated, hardened and unnatural pills. Shockingly, however, some opponents of natural medicines—possibly people aligned with Big Pharma, like the fact that some so-called "experts" have used this feature to hurt the reputation of natural remedies. A 2002 Food and Supplements Directive issued by the European Union banned producers from selling dietary supplements unless the product is first "proven as safe."

Thus, in Europe naturally grown components within supplements need to get reviewed as vigorously as high-priced, extremely dangerous drugs. Fighting mad, and rightly so, in 2005 more than one million consumers and doctors enraged by these stupid rules signed a petition calling for the elimination of such unjustifiable restrictions that prevent consumers from choosing their own natural health-care products. Following various court rulings and challenges, the European Court of Justice eventually made an idiotic final decision to uphold the restrictions—which the judges ruled was imposed for "the public good."

Generating what I proclaim as a "Nanny State gone wild," the corrupt governments of our allies and friends throughout Europe sided with greedy Big Pharma—which essentially insists that natural, safe, inexpensive and often-effective natural remedies get just as much scrutiny as extremely dangerous, high-priced drugs.

Ultimately, the demented philosophies of government bureaucrats strived to trump and destroy the rules of biology set forth by Mother Nature. Cancer and a variety of other diseases emerge as the body's natural response to toxins and biological malfunctions. To think that only "unnatural" substances like manmade drugs can effectively manage or "cure" such ailments is idiotic.

Those of us who appreciate "God" or the Devine Creator, and the scientific properties of our universe remain thankful that Mother Nature has provided humanity with a host of natural antibiotics and non-drug remedies.

Put it this way: "If and when suffering from cancer or other diseases, would you rather take only highly dangerous, synthetic and chemical-laden—sometimes poisonous—drugs made by Big Pharma as a potential cure? Or, would you like to use natural substances and foods, including those used in many supplements, vitamins, minerals and other natural, harmless substances, consistently shown by scientific research as potentially effective treatments or preventative measures? Also, would you prefer to rely on expensive pharmacies, which essentially offer no effective natural methods of detoxifying the body—a process that many scientists say, when done naturally, can go a long way in fortifying or improving the functions of the digestive system?"

Yes, as a consumer and as a patient, the choice should be yours no matter what corrupt governments or politicians that lack medical training might be telling us. For as long as people have a voice and access to critical information on this vital issue, they need to remain vigilant at encouraging the unrestricted, legal use of natural substances—particularly from plants outside the narcotics classification.

Challenges Exist in the U.S.

With crazy, poorly crafted anti-nature regulations such as those in Europe, I'm not surprised by the steady, strong number of people from around the world who visit my medical clinic in the Western United States. Although segments of the American government are corrupt as well, due partly to huge campaign donations that Big Pharma and Big Food give to some politicians, for the most part citizens of the U.S. have at least some choice on this critical issue.

The U.S. Congress passed the Dietary Supplement Health and Education Act of 1994, defining such products as "supplements" to what people eat. This makes sense, because consumers should never consider supplements as a primary food source, particularly cancer patients who have experienced extensive weight loss.

In order to be classified as a "dietary supplement," a product must contain a: mineral, vitamin, herb or an amino acid or other botanical, except tobacco. Additional factors enabling a product to enter this class can include whether the substance has historically been used as a diet supplement. In addition, within the U.S. items listed as supplements must be ingested as a liquid, powder, capsule, tablet or pill. The law requires manufacturers to label the products with the phrase "dietary supplement," while never listing the item as conventional food, and also not implying or claiming it can be used for a diet or as a meal.

Beware of the FDA

Sadly, although the ability of U.S. consumers to freely choose supplements is much better than in Europe, within the United

States the approval of such products is handled by the corrupt and inept FDA—which essentially operates within the pockets of Big Pharma.

Many of my patients, homeopaths and even standard-medicine doctors call me "the maverick doctor" for standing up against this inept federal agency. (For more specifics on this controversial issue and the ineptitude of the FDA, you can read my hot-selling 2009 book, "Your Secret to the Fountain of Youth, What they Don't Want You to Know about HGH, Human Growth Hormone."

While the criticism of my stands on this vital issue are sometimes harsh, I feel an urgent need to inform the public about how these bureaucrats are essentially "playing with the health of consumers" by favoring Big Pharma. Thankfully, however, at least for the most part within the United States, huge drug companies must first get their products approved by the FDA before those pharmaceuticals can be sold and distributed.

Chapter 25 Summary

Dietary supplements packed with vitamins, minerals and powerful antioxidant herbs can serve as formidable tools in the Forsythe Anti-Cancer Diet strategy. Supplements are not considered as foods and never should be used as replacements for meals. Effective dietary supplements can help minimize the potential inflammation caused by unhealthy fatty acids while detoxifying the body and helping cancer patients to regain strength. Rather than trying to diagnose themselves and rushing to stores to buy supplements, consumers should seek advice from licensed experienced homeopaths and dietitians. Depending on a specific patient's unique needs, some natural, generally harmless dietary supplements might do more for addressing cancers or related side effects than expensive, dangerous drugs. Although not technically foods, dietary supplements sometimes can be considered as essential for people to ingest while being treated for cancer or trying to avoid getting the disease. Sadly, in much of Europe some consumers have difficulty getting natural supplements due to harsh government regulations. In the United States, the inept and corrupt Food and Drug Administration refuses to acknowledge the anti-cancer benefits of vitamins and supplements.

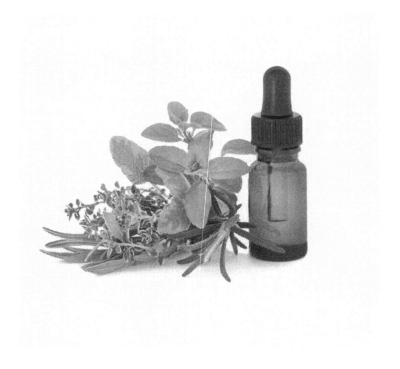

Chapter 26

Benefit
from Herbalism

Besides the potential benefits of supplements, cancer patients and people seeking to prevent the disease sometimes can generate positive results by using herbs. Within the broad spectrum of things you can eat, the beneficial use of herbs is called "herbalism."

Scientists have identified at least 12,000 plants featuring herbs ideal for use in compounds for treating diseases, according to various reports issued in 2004 and 2006, including an article in a medical chemistry magazine. Many dietary supplements are packed with herbs for this reason.

Thus, although herbs should never technically be classified as "foods that fully and wholly constitute meals," they can potentially go a long way in minimizing or controlling a variety of ailments including cancer. This is why any discussion of an effective anti-cancer diet regimen should include integral information about the benefits of herbs.

A person specializing in locating, blending or administering specific herbs is called a "herbologist." You should never first go directly to such a person in hopes of getting a thorough medical check-up or a diagnosis. Only a doctor or certified medical professional should handle those duties.

In addition, consumers hoping to seek the direct advice from a herbologist should only seek out and work with people with extensive training in this field. My clinic staff works only with qualified herbologists who serve as independent contractors. I tell patients, "Never get pushed into buying products that you don't want or that you don't need for your physical condition. If you have questions about the efficacy of a specific herb, be sure to ask me."

Homeopaths that attended medical schools often have intrinsic knowledge about herbs as well. Perhaps even more so than herbologists, a homeopath knows how the body interacts with certain herbs for long-term health benefits, battling biological invaders including cancer.

Appreciate the Unique Qualities of Herbs

Homeopaths believe that although many herbs lack essential nutrients that the body needs, these substances sometimes have the unique distinction of assisting a patient's overall natural protective mechanisms. In fact, for thousands of years physicians and medicine manufacturers have used herbs when producing drugs that eventually contain many "unnatural qualities" or overly intensified strengths. The production of heroin or other opiate-based analgesics are among examples of when manufactures refine a plant's various specific components to generate extremely high-power results. For the most part, the human body has an extremely difficult job of ingesting or processing highly concentrated drugs; intense concentrations of unnaturally mixed pharmaceutical components sometimes pose severe potential dangers including toxic overload that can lead to cancer. Largely for these reasons, doctors in recent decades have often discovered extensive tumor growths in and around the organs of people who abused narcotics in the 1960s and 1970s. Sometimes reckless and uncaring, Big Pharma puts the overall public health at risk by using chemical production processes to transform herbs into extremely dangerous, high-power and high-priced drugs.

By contrast, herbs that have not been extensively modified in a chemical-laden manufacturing process can generate fantastic benefits when carefully prescribed by a medical professional such as a homeopath for specific medical conditions.

Once again, the corrupt FDA occasionally obstructs this issue. No matter what that often-inept federal agency wants to tell the public, homeopaths know that certain herbs effectively treat specific conditions while reducing health risks, and boasting anti-inflammatory qualities beneficial in the prevention or control of cancer. Adding to the firepower, by some accounts at least 4,000 herbs or derivatives from specific foods contain polyphenol antioxidants and natural phenols. Potential benefits increase even more among herbs high in dietary fiber, sometimes called "ruffage" or "roughage," including soluble substances that assist the colon in processing gasses, and insoluble molecules that absorb water— ultimately aiding the natural biological removal of solid wastes. These attributes can boost the digestive tract's overall ability to process food, thereby clearing the way for the body to efficiently digest, absorb and use antioxidants.

Although specific, in-depth studies remain necessary on this issue, I believe that a comprehensive herb-based plan incorporated into the overall Forsythe Anti-Cancer Diet strategy can play a significant role in maintaining or improving health. Among some specific plant varieties within the dietary fiber category:

Soluble fiber: Besides nuts and almonds, often hailed for their high levels of this attribute, these many foods include sweet potatoes, onions, fruits including berries and bananas, oats, rye, barley, legumes such as beans, soybeans, and peas, and vegetables including those from roots like sweet potatoes.

Insoluble fiber: Besides wheat, corn bran and whole-grain foods, the many selections include the skins of fruits like tomatoes and kiwi, and potato skins.

Some Drug Benefits Exist

Although some drugs derived from herbs are harmful, some are beneficial in fighting cancer. A prime example here is Taxol™, a phyto-chemical that is purified and extracted from Pacific yew trees. Sometimes called by its generic name "Paclitaxel," this was discovered in 1967 by National Cancer Institute researchers. Commercially made by Bristol-Myers Squibb, this trademarked substance is sometimes used in cancer chemotherapy as a mitotic inhibitor. Taxol works to prevent cells from dividing, striving to block cancer from growing or from metastasizing. These attributes often make Taxol, sometimes sold in a new formulation called Abraxane, a formidable tool in fighting ovarian, breast and lung cancers, and advanced stages of Kaposi's sarcoma. Although Taxol is made from natural substances, it sometimes generates negative side effects similar to problems generated by typical Big Pharma pharmaceuticals. The wide range of potential problems from Taxol include brittle or thinning hair, a loss of appetite, vomiting, nausea, changes in nail color, tearing and pain lasting more than three days in the legs or joints. Even more serious side effects sometimes erupt, including dizziness or shortness of breath, fever, coughs or even infertility due to ovarian damage.

Despite its substantial potential for significant benefits, Taxol can generate far more potentially negative side effects than most herbs that are taken orally. Even more promising is the added benefit that certain herbs can be incorporated into recipes or used as "spices" in anti-cancer diets.

United States Shuns Herbs

Demographic and sociological studies consistently show that highly industrialized countries generally lack the propensity of natural herbs in their diets. Meantime, the use of beneficial natural herbs in diets is far more prevalent in less developed countries. Could this be why average life expectancies are sometimes substantially higher in less industrialized countries like Costa Rica in Central America, or certain regions of the Mediterranean where large populations suffer a low incidence of cancer?

By some accounts, including estimates by the World Health Organization, up to 80 percent of the populations throughout Asia and Africa use natural herbs as an integral part of primary health care—including for cancer treatment.

Yet you should avoid feeling "bad" or blaming yourself if you have not previously learned of the potential significant benefits of incorporating appropriate herbs into your diet. The highly industrialized mainstream medical culture in the United States, and the mega-food production processes in our country, have either purposely shunned or unintentionally avoided the significance of herbs for several generations.

Thankfully, however, due largely to the persistence of some admirable good-health organizations and limited numbers of medical professionals, steadily increasing numbers of people within our culture seem to be getting this critical message.

Although no specified, intense studies seem to show this, particularly since the beginning of the 21st Century I've seen more positive signs that the public is beginning to get a better understanding of this critical issue.

Understand Anti-Cancer Herbal Categories

Before adding herbs into their recipes and meal plans, consumers and patients wanting to boost their anti-cancer diet regimens should first understand the primary herbal categories credited with assisting the body in the control of this disease.

Prior to being harvested, many plants naturally generate various complex chemical compounds, a product of their natural metabolisms—sometimes to protect themselves from diseases or invaders. These are divided into two categories:

Primary metabolites: This sector usually generates fats and sugars found within a wide variety of plants.

Secondary metabolites: These substances often found in smaller plants than those generating primary metabolites usually perform various functions. Sometimes this generates toxins to protect a plant from predators, while other products here sometimes assist in the pollination by generating pheromones. Largely thanks to their ability to help humans, secondary metabolites serve as a primary ingredient in producing powerful drugs ranging from morphine to quinine. The many plant sources include poppy and foxglove.

Like with all substances including water and even oxygen, herbs can be toxic or even poisonous to the body when ingested in huge quantities over short periods. For this reason, you never should try to ingest huge quantities of supplements or herbs within a few hours. Rather than helping your underlying symptoms, doing so could produce a proverbial "recipe for disaster." You see, although not as dangerous overall as narcotics or Big Pharma drugs, herbs—although generally safe when used in moderation—

can generate serious health complications. Overdoses of "normally healthy" herbs seem extremely rare, at least based on the thousands of patients that I've helped.

While fully cognizant of these potential trip-ups, you can position yourself and your family for significant benefits, by incorporating appropriate amounts of herbs into your diet habits.

Alkaloids

One of the most significant segments of the various chemical compounds that plants generate is "alkaloids." This sector includes some of the most powerful anti-cancer attributes from among at least five primary herb-based chemical compound categories.

Although the mainstream standard medical industry blatantly ignores this fact, helpful and natural alkaloids are produced in abundance worldwide by plants and animals. Scientists have found these secondary metabolites from a variety of sources including fungi and bacteria. People eager to prevent cancer or other diseases often appreciate the fact that although many alkaloid chemical compounds contain toxins as a protective measure, scientists have developed methods of isolating the beneficial qualities of these same substances—especially when producing various helpful medications.

However, once again caution also becomes necessary because some alkaloids are used as recreational drugs, or even for dangerous "entheogen" rituals performed by various religions and spiritual organizations. These range from highly potent peyote to extremely dangerous psilocybin mushrooms. Understandably, no certified herbologist or homeopath should ever recommend or administer such substances to people, even as supposed "foods or supplements" touted as cancer treatments. If and when you ever get encouraged to eat highly toxic substances, immediately avoid the person who recommended them and seek help elsewhere right away.

Many foods and herbs within this sector have psychoactive properties that can seriously alter the thought process, causing horrific hallucinations and perhaps even generating permanent brain damage, liver destruction or death. This emerges as so dangerous that many so-called herbs within the alkaloid class are listed by the federal government and most states as felony-class substances. One of the most dangerous is LSD, derived primarily from Convolvulaceae, an alkaloid within the "ergoline family" gleaned from certain species of fungi and even various types of vines.

Due primarily to the extremely power attributes of alkaloids, Big Pharma often uses them to produce some of the strongest and potentially the most dangerous drugs for treatment of a wide variety of specific ailments. One of the most notorious still used for specific medical purposes is cocaine, famous as a local anesthetic and stimulant. Quinidine is used for anti-arrhythmia and ephedrine is used for asthma, just some of the many examples of using powerful alkaloids for legitimate medical purposes.

While careful to avoid these types of dangerous alkaloids, although they come from "natural plants," you also can rest assured that many alkaloids are healthful and often recommended as regular anti-cancer diet components.

Alkaloids that Fight Cancer

At least two alkaloids are frequently used by physicians to fight tumors, but they are not found often enough to provide adequate cancer-fighting food sources. Manufacturers can only isolate and produce limited amounts of Vinblastine for treating a variety of cancers, primarily of the breast, lung, head and neck, plus Hodgkin's Lymphoma. Derived from a Madagascar periwinkle, the "vinca rosea," also called "Catharanthus ruseus," the plant forms this substance by joining two alkaloids. Doctors sometimes use Vinblastine as part of chemotherapy regimens. The second anti-cancer alkaloid treatment involves Vincristine, often effective in preventing tumor cells from dividing—thereby preventing the disease from growing and spreading. Both of these drugs have been around for almost 50 years, and are called "spindle disruptors," as they interfere with the cancer cell division into two daughter cells.

Despite the potential effectiveness of Vinblastine and Vincristine, these substances are only available intravenously. So, patients should avoid any attempt to eat the rare plants used to make those medications. Vincristine, also from the Madagascar periwinkle, can cause death or neurotoxicity if administered incorrectly.

Primary Chemical Compounds

Besides alkaloids, the three other primary chemical compounds deserve mention, some already referred to briefly in previous pages. They are:

Polyphenols: Most often purple, these usually have strong antioxidant and anti-cancer attributes. These include: the tannins from tea; isoflavones from certain grapes; and phytoestrogens from soy. Isoflavones can efficiently trap singlet oxygen, an attribute often credited with lowering the dangers of breast cancer. Although often considered as "anti-nutritional," meaning that they sometimes interfere with the body's absorption of nutrients, tannins may help reverse certain toxic overloads that otherwise could lead to cancer. Also deemed helpful in protecting the kidneys, tannins have been credited with fighting harmful bacteria, viruses and even some parasites. Foods containing tannins include pomegranate, persimmons, nuts and berries. More specifically, within the herb classification, other potentially effective tannin sources include cinnamon, vanilla, curcumin, cloves and tarragon. In addition, phytoestrogens from soy within the polyphenol classification play an integral function as a female sex hormone. Sometimes called "dietary estrogens" when initially produced outside the body, phytoestrogens come from a wide variety of foods. Besides oilseeds and nuts, some of the most common sources include cereals and breads derived from soy, meat products and legumes. Scientists say phytoestrogen levels vary among foods, but they're often highest in soybean. Other common sources include oats, beans, barley, alfalfa and carrots, plus yams, beans, wheat berries and sesame seeds. Some consumers might be surprised to discover that phytoestrogens are sometimes found in licorice root, mint, beer, bourbon and even coffee. Various recent studies including a "life science" report indicate that phytoestrogens may help protect men against prostate cancer. Separate studies at Cornell and in Ontario, Canada, generate inclusive results on whether phytoestrogens cause or prevent breast cancer in women. However, some reports indicate that women who've suffered from current or past breast cancers risk getting tumors when taking soy products. Overall, researchers seem to believe more study is needed to determine the potential dangers or benefits of isoflavones such as those from soybeans, impacting potential breast cancers in women. This remains a gray area in both breast and prostate cancers.

Glycosides: Also within the alkaloid class of primary chemical compounds, these molecules have a unique ability within living organisms to activate specific enzymes, breaking away certain sugars. This unique quality might play an integral role in fighting cancer. Remember, as stated earlier, researchers know that cancers thrive on simple sugars. This also emerges as a primary reason why glycosides are often used for the production of medications. Additional benefits emerge when taking into account the fact that poisons often bind to sugar molecules as they're naturally removed as waste from the body. Thanks to this unique quality, doctors sometimes administer or recommend glycosides. Scientists believe that besides having certain pain-killing attributes, glycosides can play a formidable role as an effective anti-inflammatory— an essential role in fighting cancer. Some glycosides have "cyanogenic" attributes, meaning that they produce toxic hydrogen cyanide as the molecule's sugar portion gets released. Besides almonds, other foods within this class include cherries, crabapples, apples, plumbs, apricots, raspberries and peaches. According to some published reports, cyanogenic glycosides once had a reputation for having significant anti-cancer attributes, but various studies since then may have debunked such claims.

Terpenes: One of the most diverse and largest classes of chemical compounds, or "organic compounds," of herbs, this segment is derived primarily from conifers. Mostly large, cone-bearing trees, these cover a wide variety of species such as junipers, firs, cypresses, hemlocks, spruces and even redwoods. By some accounts, these cover at least 550 species that stem from eight overall categories. While their major products include turpentine and resin, scientists insist that almost every living creature has essential biosynthetic building blocks of terpenes. In fact, many fragrances from perfumes and flavors from foods come from the essential oils found in terpenes and terpenoids. Terpene serves as a significant source of Vitamin A, and this segment also covers the vital antioxidant carotenoid category mentioned earlier. At least ten classifications of terpenes generate a wide variety of chemical substances, some that may have anti-cancer or anti-oxidant attributes. These include retinol.

Warning: Anti-Cancer Herbs Face Extinction

An urgent trend has been widely ignored by the mainstream news media, the fact that several vital plants that produce herbs effective in fighting cancer face a risk of extinction. The rapid worldwide spread of deforestation and over-harvesting threaten:

Yew trees: From conifers once prevalent in their native Pacific Northwest, a region of North America, this species grew naturally from Central California all the way northward to the southernmost areas of Alaska. The most prevalent areas have included huge swaths of south central Idaho, and portions of British Columbia in Canada. Often growing from 10 meters to 15 meters, this evergreen tree sometimes reaches up to 20 meters, particularly within gullies or protected areas like parks. This tree has been the primary source for Paclitaxel, sometimes sold under the trademark Taxol™, often effective in preventing the spread of cancer cells following chemotherapy. Paclitaxel has been used in the treatment of head and neck, breast, ovarian, prostate and lung cancers, plus Kaposi's Sarcoma. Scientists spent many years of intense research on how to most effectively harvest the effective ingredients of yew trees, until finally fine-tuning the harvesting process in the early 1990s. But controversy erupted amid concerns of over-harvesting this herb in the Pacific Northwest. According to the "Florida State University Research and Review," an improved process that increased yield cleared the way to begin manufacturing in Ireland in 1992, using needles of European yew. Now, using technology developed by Phyton Biotech, Inc., manufacturers use endrophytic fungus when making Paclitaxel in large fermentation tanks.

Magnolias: According to some reports, including stories

in BBC News, more than half of magnolias worldwide have disappeared. This loss could emerge as significant. For more than 5,000 years beginning in China, physicians have used herbs from magnolias to fight cancer, dementia and heart disease. Biologists have identified at least 210 species of this flowering plant, found primarily across East and Southeast Asia, the West Indies, South America, Central America and North America. According to a 2009 article by the National Institutes of Health, honokiol found within magnolias have anti-tumor and anti-inflammatory qualities. These have been used as a component in Asian herbal teas.

Chapter 26 Summary

Many natural herbs, some included in dietary supplements, are powerful and formidable as antioxidants. Bowing to the wishes of Big Pharma and ignoring patients' needs, standard oncologists consider Herbalism as "quackery." Although more study needs to be done on this critical issue, incorporating herbs into the overall Forsythe Anti-Cancer Diet strategy can play a critical role in maintaining or improving health. Some herbs are used to make drugs helpful in fighting cancer. Highly industrialized countries like the United States use effective anti-cancer herbs less than societies in relatively poor undeveloped countries. Although natural, herbs can be highly toxic in excessive doses over short periods. Alkaloids are among the most powerful anti-cancer herbs, but also are used in producing extremely dangerous narcotics like LSD. Two specific types of alkaloids, have been helpful in fighting cancer, but they're not found in enough abundance to use as food. Three other herb-based chemical compounds besides alkaloids have been helpful in fighting cancer; polyphenols from soybeans, oats, beans, barley, alfalfa, carrots and other foods; glycosides with a unique ability to break away sugars, making them ideal in the production of medications; and Terpenes, from cone-bearing trees, significant sources of Vitamin A. Some plants that feature anti-cancer herbs face potential extinction in the wild, including yew trees primarily in the U.S. Pacific Northwest and wild-growing magnolia species worldwide.

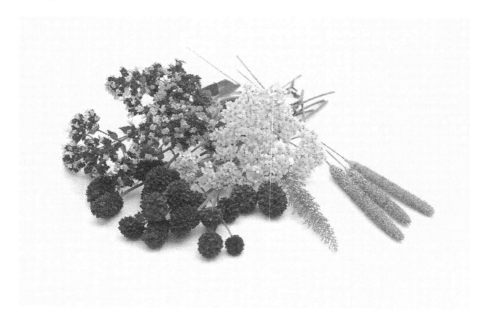

Chapter 27

Processed Food
Dangers

A brief but urgent discussion on the dangers of processed foods becomes necessary in any anti-cancer diet, especially since we've consistently urged patents to avoid them.

Some consumers and patients still remain confused about what precisely is a "processed food," and why they are dangerous. So, an explanation becomes vital.

In summary, a processed food is any meal or snack produced en mass for a variety of reasons, which for each specific product can hinge on some or all of these factors:

Efficiency: Farmers, distributors, stores and in some cases restaurants want to get meals, specific foods or snacks to consumers as quickly and efficiently as possible.

Cut costs: Rather than compiling and sending food at high cost in huge bulky crates or boxes, food processors strive to cut expenses as much as possible to increase profit.

Packaging: Quickly made packages, sometimes aluminum and "cheap" plastics, enable shippers and stores to put high quantities of products in tight, efficient spaces—ultimately reducing costs.

Preservatives: Foods in cans, bottles and plastics are sometimes loaded with dangerous levels of chemical preservatives that might increase cancer dangers. Manufacturers use preservatives in hopes of increasing a product's shelf life, the time expected for the food to spoil—a date at which the item is no longer deemed salable.

Salts: Often as an additive, preservative, and to enhance flavors, many manufacturers started packing salt into snacks— particularly potato chips and nuts. Besides leading to arterial problems, excessive consumption of salts can lead to high blood pressure and ultimately strokes.

Food types: The previously mentioned processing features impact consumers buying many types of foods ranging from candy, soft drinks, juice, fruits, vegetables, dairy products and nutty snacks. Microwavable meals in tightly fit plastic containers might seem like the most obvious offenders. Some crops offered in the so-called "natural" produce section also might be considered "processed"—at least in the sense that they're delivered and sold in plastics that have been zipped through automated high-production mechanical systems.

All these factors work individually and in combinations to ultimately make foods that homeopaths and dietitians often considered as "unhealthy." Studies seem to vary widely on potential dangers. Among key factors to consider: Do results or findings vary, based on who conducts this research? Do consumer-oriented organizations get results indicating certain fast foods pose dangers, while research done by big-food processors show minimal or no potential health problems?

Well, from my view as a medical professional, there seems little doubt that the high consumption of "preservative" chemicals—especially over extended periods lasting many months or years—very likely emerges as a major contributor to the growing cancer problem in the USA.

From everything you've discovered so far here, the dangers of potential bodily invaders should seem evident, particularly plastics, aluminums, chemicals and other toxins—many from processed food. Meats and cheese, particularly those sold in plastics or Styrofoam, might have been processed in massive quantities. Despite these potential dangers, the nation's consumption of processed foods has skyrocketed, especially starting in the late 1940s after the end of World War II.

Those in the Baby Boom generation born from 1946 through 1964, are only now beginning to suffer from increasingly high cancer rates among their age group. Particularly within the United States, this was history's first generation to become consistently exposed to processed foods in massive, non-stop quantities on an almost daily basis. Much of this began with TV dinners that initially were on the market on a fairly limited basis, before booming on a widespread scale from the late '60s onward.

Sadly, today the vast majority of foods available in grocery stores are processed partly in order to get products to consumers fast on a widespread scale. These quick-to-market tactics have spilled over into everything from most ice creams to plastic-wrapped cake snacks.

Herein emerges a significant reason why I sometimes caution patients to become wary when they see package labels that boast of containing "only natural ingredients." Although a food might contain such substances, the process of quickly formulating and packaging those substances might have made the item a processed food. Prime examples sometimes involve so-called natural spices sold en masse for eventual use when cooking meals on stovetops or ovens. These entail everything from brownie mixes to gravies, macaroni and cheese, cake mixes, meat spices that sometimes contain trans fats, preservatives and unhealthful fillers while sold in plastics or aluminum. An added problem unrelated to potentially carcinogenic foods develops, the increasingly complex issues of food packaging that ultimately contaminates or loads landfills.

As a consumer, you need to take an active and diligent role in striving to avoid processed foods, while cognizant that your long-term survival—and that of your family—could very well hinge upon steering clear of such items as much as possible.

Chapter 27 Summary

Processed foods impose numerous potentially carcinogenic dangers. To cut costs, maximize efficiencies and improve storage of foods, major manufacturers and distributors zip crops through packaging machines that cover products in dangerous plastics and metals like aluminum—while also jamming carcinogenic preservatives into the meals.

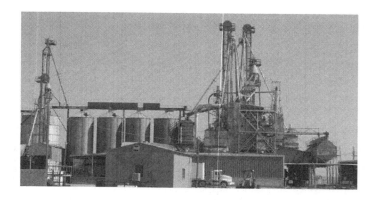

Chapter 28

Urgent:
Boost Your Immunity

Did you know that a weak immunity can emerge as a key factor in eventually triggering cancer or clearing the way for the disease to spread within the body?

Well, don't feel discouraged if you never knew this. I've helped thousands of cancer patients previously were unaware that their immune systems were too weak prior to receiving treatments elsewhere. Luckily, specific foods can play an integral role in boosting the body's ability to fight cancer and other disease.

Before learning what specific foods sometimes help this, it's essential to know the basics of how a typical person naturally fights disease. Biologically, this happens in two ways that sometimes interact or compliment each other:

Innate: Cells within the body aggressively attack invaders including pathogens, bacteria or toxins likely to trigger cancer. Scientists believe the innate or "cellular immune system" battles virtually all substances that the body considers as foreign.

Adaptive: This highly specialized but natural process essentially has a "memory" of previous invaders. Once your body has been attacked by bacteria or viruses, such as specific influenza strains suffered at a young age, the cellular system develops highly specialized soldiers highly effective at battling any future barrage by similar usurpers. Thankfully, an identical invader fails at creating serious or even fatal damage during subsequent attacks, in some cases even cancer.

When deciding which foods will best assist your innate and adaptive immune systems, your homeopath or dietitian also needs to consider what impact the meals likely would generate within the body's organ systems that specialize in fighting invaders.

Many everyday people know that bone marrow plays an essential role in immunity, creating critical cells necessary for fighting harmful bacteria and certain diseases. Yet, at least within the overall public mindset, much less credit seems to go to three other primary organ systems. These are: the spleen, which helps the body keep critical immune-boosting cells, while filtering blood; the thymus, which generates the critical T-cells, "killers" designed to seek out and destroy invading bacteria and cancer; and the lymph nodes, essentially storage facilities that contain the "factories that make the body's vital weapons of war"—proteins that render foreign cells as inert. The lymph notes also process lymph fluid. Think of the lymph fluid transportation system as a deceptive executioner, sending invaders to the nodes where the attackers get destroyed.

Good Foods Play a Critical Role

Abundant or at least adequate levels of specific nutritious foods are necessary on a continuous basis for the body to enable these various immunological systems to work efficiently enough for maintaining good health.

You see, the body continually makes immune-boosting cells. But these same molecular structures that people need to survive

268

have extremely short life spans.

Thus, without adequate nutrition and antioxidants that the body can readily and efficiently absorb, the body fails to make enough protective cells. When the continuous production of these helpful biological structures dips to critically low levels for extended periods, disease such as cancer develops. Ultimately, unless corrective measures are taken at this urgent juncture, death occurs among numerous cells and possibly the end of the person's life. Everything within the individual's overall biological structure starts coming to a halt if and when the following factors come to play— in some cases due at least partly to an inadequate diet:

Macrophages: This specific type of white blood cell steadily beings to—or fully loses—its ability to perform two essential functions that they normally perform with ease. First, macrophages start losing their ability to detect invaders. Secondly, and just as destructive, these same cells also lose their abilities to annihilate or scavenge attackers.

Dendrite: Sometimes called "dendritic" cells, these are the specialized macrophages that serve as "scout soldiers," traveling throughout the body to find specific types of invaders including cancer cells. The moment a dendrite cell finds an attacker, the dendrite immediately makes a record of this critical discovery. Right away, a healthy dendrite cell rushes back to the home base to relay this critical information necessary for survival.

Lymphocyte: Commonly called "white blood cells," these warriors rush to the battlefield right after receiving the critical go-to-war messages from dendrite cells. Two types of specialized lymphocyte cells enter the fray, a critical phase in determining whether the body is able to adequately fight and prevent the spread of cancer or other invaders. The initial first wave usually involves T-helper cells, specialized lymphocytes that also essentially serve as "war generals" and other top military commanders—working together to develop the most effective battle plan. As seasoned warriors, the T-helper cells determine if the immune system has previously responded to similar invaders. When that's the case T-helper cells summon their second-phase reinforcements, the killer T-cells that relentlessly strive to obliterate the enemy.

Natural killers: Critical to the innate immune system, within people who have healthy immunity thanks in part to good nutrition, natural killer cells sometimes called "NK" stream into the forefront. Natural killers strive to come to the rescue in instances of perceived new threats, instances where the body fails to recognize the attackers as previous invaders. For a T-cell to work effectively against a particular invader the body must have had previous experience battling that type of invader. By contrast, natural killers are much different. The NK go after any perceived invader, although the same natural killers lack previous experience handling those specific situations. Due to these unique characteristics, the natural killers often end up working the hardest and most diligently at battling cancer. The disease often evolves or strives to change as part of its own protective and attacking mechanisms.

Suppressor T-cells: After the initial fray, these specialized immunity cells strive to keep everything on an even keel, essentially calming the situation. When healthy, in part due to an adequate nutritious diet and the ingestion of antioxidants, suppressor T-cells strive to keep your immune system in balance. Essentially, these serve as the body's way to keep from overreacting. In a way, the suppressor T-cells are like coaches at the corner of a boxing ring. A seasoned, wise and well-informed coach discourages his boxer from flailing away wildly and furiously without any effective game plan. Otherwise, the fighter is likely to expend far too much energy, become overly exhausted and eventually lose the long-term battle. Well, for fights involving killer T-cells and natural killers, the suppressor T-cells perform an essential role in preventing fights from getting out of hand. Otherwise the body likely would push its immune system into overdrive, a tenuous situation that likely would result in the complete shutdown of this entire structure.

Eat Specific Foods to Boost Immunity

Any person who fails to eat adequate amounts of healthy, unprocessed foods is essentially encouraging the immune system to weaken—potentially resulting in cancer. You see, a vitamin deficiency in any area of the body can eventually trigger a cascading or domino effect, ultimately leading to the disease.

Prime examples here involve toxins mentioned earlier that damage the liver, or the inadequate ingestion of oils critical in keeping that organ system clean enough to efficiently operate. Thus, in order to boost or maintain immunity, an effective Forsythe Anti-Cancer Diet regimen requires:

Beverages: To maintain good health and ensure optimal immune functions, many scientists and nutritional experts say you should drink at least half of a gallon of healthy beverages daily. This means at least 64 ounces of fluid. Some health professionals suggest drinking at least eight 8-ounce glasses of water, consumed throughout the day. This must be toxin-free, purified or filtered water, which also should serve as the primary ingredient for green or herbal teas.

White sugar: As stated earlier, cancer essentially loves and thrives upon white sugar due largely to the energy that such foods provide. But consumers, and particularly people wanting to prevent cancer or to control the disease, also need to know that white sugar decreases the body's ability to make its natural immune-boosting antibodies. Compounding these issues, some scientists also believe that sugars at least temporarily impede the ability of white blood cells to battle harmful pathogens like cancer. Adding to these difficulties, critical fatty acids lose their ability to effectively protect the digestive system and internal organs. As if these problems weren't already enough, immunity can get weakened or compromised when sugars generate an unhealthful or dangerous imbalance among minerals. The body has a relatively easy time processing simple carbohydrates, but complex high-sugar foods do quite the opposite—causing severe and almost immediate negative impacts on immunity shortly after digestion.

Understand and Use Whey

Many consumers have never heard of "whey," considered by many homeopaths and dietitians as among the most powerful immune-boosting foods. Manufacturers indirectly create whey as a byproduct of the casein- and cheese-making process.

Also a strong anti-oxidant and sometimes called "milk serum," whey is generally healthful to the immune system when regularly eaten in recommended quantities. Technically, whey is formed during the intentional curdling process of separating cheese from milk. By contrast, custards are created when the curdling is unintentional, byproducts of various cooking or mixing processes. Whey products are produced in two forms:

Sweet whey: Created when producing cheeses with complex rennet enzymes, particularly Swiss cheese and cheddar.

Sour whey: This forms as a byproduct when making cottage cheese and other acid cheeses.

Whey has much different benefits when used directly by consumers and manufacturers. For food makers, whey is necessary for making brown cheeses and ricotta. More importantly from the perspective of consumers and people on anti-cancer diets, whey is often an excellent nutritional supplement. Bodybuilders like whey thanks largely to its protein-packed natural ability to nourish the body and particularly the muscles, eliminating any foolish effort to rely on extremely dangerous steroids.

Whey is often sold as various separate popular drinks ranging from "wine" to "sack," particularly in Europe. Consumers sometimes buy it as a butter or cream.

The powdered form of whey sold in some major U.S. department stores gives added benefit to people trying to lose weight or to fortify their immune systems—particularly for anti-cancer or immune-boosting regimens.

When sold in stores, most whey protein comes in powder form so that consumers can easily mix it into smoothies or health-oriented juicers. Some dietitians insist that consumers only buy whey that says "cold processed" or "un-denatured" on labels. This is critical to check because the denaturation food-making process essentially robs food of nutrients.

Remember, like all other antioxidant foods or other meals included within the immune-boosting category, whey should never be considered a "be-all, and end-all" part of treatment or prevention for cancer patients. Even so, whey can potentially generate formidable benefits due to its unique qualities, primarily:

Protein: The proteins or essential amino acids within whey can be isolated, power-packed with the energy necessary to help give your body a fighting chance or to help the immune system. Technically, these are called "whey proteins," labeled by scientists as globular proteins.

Lactose: Although a potentially strong food for your immune system, whey should be avoided by lactose-intolerant people. In most forms whey contains high amounts of lactose. The potential dangers can multiply for lactose-intolerant individuals because dried whey contains up to 70 percent lactose when used as a common food additive. These amounts sometimes vastly exceed levels that lactose-intolerant people can tolerate. Lactose is a sugar from milk or from various dairy products made from milk. The many adverse symptoms of lactose intolerance can potentially exacerbate or worsen health issues already suffered by cancer patients. Frequent ailments suffered by lactose intolerant people include flatulence, diarrhea, abdominal bloating, vomiting, nausea and a "rumbling stomach" condition that doctors call borborygmus—accompanied by a rumbling or gurgling noise.

Vitamins and minerals: Whey products are packed with these vital substances, good for healthy people but particularly for those seeking to boost immunity.

Added benefits: Whey supplements can help regulate spikes in blood sugar, the same conditions that—when left unchecked—can either contribute to the development of cancer or counteract the ability of white blood cells to effectively attack invaders.

Boosting overall immunity even further, when eaten in concentrated form whey protein can boost the body's internal production of the natural antioxidant glutathione, at least according to some studies. Additional research also indicates that whey contains strong levels of amino acid cysteine, a possible weapon against breast cancer.

Eat Healthy Chlorella

These miniscule single-cell algae have been shown by numerous studies as a potentially powerful ally in helping the body maintain effective immunity.

While generally considered by some researchers as a "whole food supplement," chlorella is often sold as a tablet, liquid or powder. Consumers can often find chlorella in the natural supplement sections of major department stores or at specialized nutrition stores. It's also available via herbologists and homeopaths, some who insist that their product is far more powerful and potent than so-called cheap, common brands.

From my view, most chlorella products have significant potential health benefits, particularly those that have not been embedded into other foods.

When people regularly eat pure chlorella in sufficient quantities the potential befits can include:

Immunity: Stimulate the immunity, strengthening the body's ability to fight cancer or ailments and conditions that eventually lead to the disease.

Detoxify: Remove harmful invaders including bacteria or possibly metals from the body, thereby lessening the overwork of the various natural immune systems.

Energy: A boost in overall physical energy, once again clearing the way for the body to naturally and effectively fight or prevent cancerous tumors or other invaders.

Good cells: Some researchers insist that when consumed and fully absorbed in ideal conditions, the body actually boosts its natural production of helpful white blood cells.

Once again, as with all apparent anti-oxidants and reported immune boosters, I urge patients and consumers to avoid fully relying on chlorella. Using just one antioxidant or immune booster, particularly without the guidance of a health professional is a recipe for disaster. Nonetheless, through many years of direct interaction with patients I've found that chlorella, especially blue-green chlorella, can play a definitive role in boosting or maintaining immunity.

What are Succulent Plants?

For thousands of years, health professionals and native physicians have touted the benefits of aloe—the most famous "aloe vera." As an overall class, aloe is derived from at least 500 species of what biologists call "succulent plants."

Although widely popular for many generations among advocates of natural foods, the widespread use of the term "aloe vera" seemed non-existent—until the late 1980s when I started seeing more medical reports on its numerous apparent benefits. Among its most significant attributes that some researchers claimed to find in laboratory studies:

Shrinkage: A reduction in the total mass of tumors, experienced by cancerous rats that started eating aloe.

Metastases: The spread of the disease within the body slowed or stopped, giving hope to cancer patients everywhere.

While some health-food advocates or producers of so-called good foods occasionally tout their aloe-based products as "secret" or a "miracle," I often caution patients to remain fully aware that no known cure-all exists. Nonetheless, as with chlorella, at least based on my experience, the healthful use of aloe seems to help work wonders in the recovery process or at the very least in health-maintenance efforts. According to many publications, like chlorella, aloe seems to energize immunity by increasing white blood cell production.

Found in many health food stores or often within over-the-counter medicine or supplement sections of department stores, aloe is usually sold as a concentrated powder, gel or even a juice.

Many consumers apparently learn about the apparent wonders of aloe vera or other aloe products via TV or radio infomercials. Lots of these advertisements feature doctors, patients or even representatives from manufacturers. At least within this big-pitch realm, just about every company offering such products seems to insist its aloe is the best, "most powerful on the planet. Ours was specially-formulated over a period of many years by a widely acclaimed team of specialized scientific researchers."

But which product is truly best, and how should you know where to purchase such items? Before answering these questions, these are just some of the initial queries that you should pose:

Costs: When considering competing items, you might discover that both products have the same ingredients, primarily aloe or aloe vera. A particularly aloe product pitched on TV might cost far more than a competitor's item advertised on the radio. Rest assured, from my experience higher-costing aloe products are not necessarily more effective.

Free: Lots of infomercials tout aloe vera products, or even supplements that also contain chlorella, as "free" for your first doses so that you can "just try it with no obligation." After that, unless you cancel, in many instances your credit card will automatically get charged for subsequent deliveries.

Only shipping: For many health supplements, particularly aloe or chlorella, we're told that the "first order is 100-percent free" or at a significant price reduction, while "all you pay for is shipping." All along, I suspect, the actual mailing charge eventually imposed on consumers is at inflated rates—immediately putting the seller at a break-even level or perhaps a minimal-profit mode.

Before rushing to buy from such sales via phone or by Websites, you might save more by first checking at your local store, or getting advice from your homeopath or dietitian. This makes sense. After all, why go through all the ordering hassles and expenses, when you could simply make a purchase while you're at the supermarket or your health professional's office?

Perhaps even more important, you should first get a thorough medical exam and a recommendation on a product—if any—from a certified health professional. Through the years I've learned that certain cheap store-bought products emerge as ineffective while others seem to work fine. The best results often emerge directly from your chosen homeopath or herbologist.

Lots of the time, as long as you're already scheduled to see these professionals anyway, during or immediately after these visits some actually give "free" samples that enable you to avoid shipping costs. This becomes an ideal way to discover if the product works.

Using this to your advantage, keep in mind that some producers of herbs and natural plants such as aloe and chlorella also give occasional complimentary samples to qualified medical professionals—who in turn can sometimes pass these products on to patients.

As an added benefit, aloe, chlorella and most natural herbs are far less expensive than pharmaceuticals made by Big Pharma. A single bottle of many dozens or even hundreds of natural supplement capsules sometimes equals the fee that the drug industry charges for just a single pill. Yes, "going natural" is almost always far less expensive, far more healthful and much less dangerous.

Employ Other Immunity Tactics

Other potentially effective natural immune-boosting strategies include eating ample garlic, striving to reduce stress, and checking with your health professional on the potential use of immune-balancing herbs like cat's claw and astragalus. Among the beneficial attributes of these herbs listed by homeopaths and herbologists:

Astragalus: Scientists have identified more than 3,000 species worldwide, many from small shrubs derived from within the legume species that range from alfalfa, carob, soy, peanuts and many other foods. Mostly found within temperate climates in the Northern Hemisphere, astragalus comes from a specific subset of legume—the fabaceae species of flowering plants. As a sub-family or subset of legume, fabaceae is found worldwide. Numerous studies indicate that although astragalus does not directly attack cancer. Yet it's credited with sharply boosting immunity, thereby serving as a potential tool in a patient's overall recovery regimen. The Chinese have known this for many hundreds or perhaps thousands of years, using astragalus as a natural herbal medicine. An active natural ingredient within astragalus, cycloastragenol, has been deemed so powerful that scientists in 2009 studied its potential uses in battling infections usually blamed on aging and chronic diseases including AIDS, according to a United Press International story. At least according to a 2008 article in the "Journal of Immunology," some researchers concluded that the immune cells age slower when boosted with cycloastragenol. If true, this means that cancer patients who consistently include astragalus in their diets while under a homeopath's care may have the added benefit of boosting their immunity for the longer term. All along, however, scientists have noted numerous potential negative side effects from astragalus, including the possibility of rising blood pressure and increased blood sugar levels, according to the National Center for Complimentary and Alternative Medicine. Complicating the situation further, the same organization reports that it has discovered some specific astragalus species that are toxic. Largely for these reasons, patients should always ask their homeopaths if the specific astragalus that they recommend comes from a species deemed safe or non-toxic.

Cat's Claw: Featuring claw-shaped thorns, this woody

vine from tropical rainforests in Central America and South America, sometimes called un de gato, has been used for a wide variety of purposes among practitioners of alternative medicine. While homeopaths sometimes recommend cat's claw for a wide variety of intestinal ailments, it's also deemed by many natural medicine practitioners as an excellent anti-cancer agent, and as an antioxidant that seems to work as an anti-inflammatory. Although cat's claw has a wide variety of other apparent or reported benefits ranging from aiding with prostate conditions to chronic fatigue, some patients might suffer from allergic reactions—particularly those sensitive to herb or food products derived from within the Rubiaceae species of flowering plants that includes coffee, gallium or "bedstraw" used in producing some red dyes, and Rubia. Besides the potential for inflammation of the kidneys, other reported possible allergic symptoms can include rashes and itching. In addition, patients should be aware that numerous other types of plants also are called "cat's claw," but those are a completely different and unrelated species.

Despite the potential adverse effects of astragalus and cat's claw, they can emerge as formidable immune boosters when ingested under the care of a certified health professional.

Stress Reduction

Another key strategy in boosting immunity involves reducing stress. While voluminous books and films have been produced on how to reduce stress, here is a brief basic summary of potential strategies:

Allergies: Get a medical test designed specifically to determine any allergies to food or medicines, and then remove those substances from your routine. Besides obvious ailments or negative symptoms, some meals might actually increase your stress levels.

Vitamin deficiency: The same medical exam also should determine if your body lacks adequate levels of specific vitamins. Such deficiencies occasionally lead to stress within the body, conditions that sometimes weaken overall immunity.

Interactions: In addition, your physician also should strive to determine if you suffer from elevated stress due to adverse interactions among foods that you eat and medicines or herbs that you take on a regular basis.

Yoga: There are many types of this relaxation, stretching, mind-management and overall health lifestyle. You should consider seeking lessons for or the regular use of specific yoga routines that professionals deem as excellent stress reducers.

Biofeedback: Using machines to monitor your body's moment-to-moment functions, giving continual readouts indicating everything from heart rate and breathing levels to muscle tension. Under the guidance of professionals skilled at this genre, under ideal conditions a patient learns to breath well, relax the entire body and to calm the mind—ultimately minimizing overall stress.

Massage: Some people also consider massage therapy as highly relaxing, greatly reducing anxiety and overall stress levels.

Along with exercise, these are just some of the many potential stress-reduction techniques that you can consider. While most of these strategies do not specifically stem from food choices, everyone eager to benefit from Forsythe Anti-Cancer Diet strategies needs to realize that "who we are is far more than merely what we eat."

Remember that although a sensible diet can and often does help to control or prevent cancer, lifestyle choices and our overall environments also play critical roles. Thus, in a sense trying to cure or minimize the disease merely via diet strategies alone would be the proverbial equivalent of trying to drive a car without the benefit of a steering wheel. Throughout life we often have the ability to choose from among many diverse paths or potential possibilities. And, the anti-cancer choices that we make every day entail far more than just food selections.

Estimate Your Own Immune Function

While also careful to get adequate sleep and moderate exercise—both of them often excellent immune boosters and stress reducers, many people can get a basic idea of their own immune function without first getting a check-up. Remember, you should never under any circumstances attempt to serve as your own physician or try to diagnose your medical condition. Nonetheless, through many years of observing patients, I've identified numerous "warning signs" that you can watch for, possible signals that your body might lack sufficient immunity.

For instance, do your lymph glands such as the organs in your neck or armpits seem overly sensitive or swollen? Perhaps you get far too many colds, many more instances of the flu or continually runny noses than most of your friends, relatives or acquaintances. Possible warning signs can include the continual re-emergence of long-term negative health conditions like nagging cold sores or pesky reoccurrences of genital herpes symptoms that you initially suffered many years ago. Perhaps just as distressing, do you always seem to suffer from some sort of chronic infection?

While only a certified medical professional can make a reliable diagnosis, you should consider such conditions as essentially "green traffic lights, signaling for you to get a check-up right away." To do otherwise, even though you might feel relatively healthy overall, could end up being to foolishly ignore what your body is struggling to tell you. Remember, your body is a part of nature, and you should view such apparent warning signs as if distant clouds that might signal a fast-approaching horrific storm that doesn't care who it destroys or how.

Chapter 28 Summary

Specific foods can help rekindle, boost or fortify the body's immunity, which can lead to cancer if weakened. Without antioxidants and adequate nutrition, the body's various types of protective white blood cells that shield and fight foreign substances could lose their abilities to respond well to various threats of cancer. To boost immunity, drink at least 64 ounces of non-toxic fluids daily, avoid eating white sugars, and consider adding protein-packed whey to your diet to maximize bodily strength and energy. Studies show a single-cell algae, chlorella— sometimes found in supplement form, helps anti-cancer regimens by boosting immunity, detoxifying the body, providing energy and increasing the production of helpful white blood cells. Other immune-boosting herbs include: astragalus, derived from many small shrubs, alfalfa, carob, soy, peanuts and other foods; and cat's claw, derived from a woody vine from rainforests in Central America and South America. People also can boost immunity by reducing their stress, using a variety of methods that include eating adequate vitamins, exercise, message, biofeedback and getting proper medical attention for allergies.

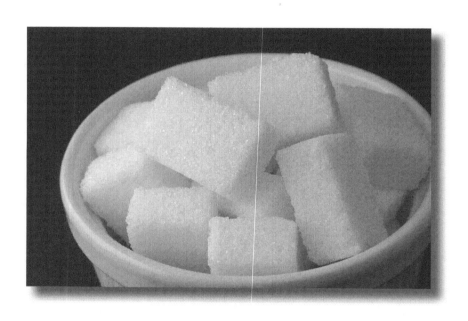

Chapter 29

Reduce
Simple Sugars

Throughout every phase of the instruction process, as you've already seen here multiple times, we've continually told patients of the urgent need to avoid simple sugars—sometimes known as "white sugar."

Yet for many people, especially those with a sweet tooth that brings a penchant for sugary treats and carbohydrates, the questions become: "How can I possibly stop eating sugar? What sugars are bad and which are good? I know sugars are often a primary cause of cancer or a blockade in controlling the disease, but does that mean that I have to suffer throughout the remainder of my life eating nothing but bland food?"

Well, before giving direct and appropriate responses, a need to reiterate this: Not only do high levels of sugar lead to obesity and its resulting health complications. Excessive amounts of this food actually encourage and help tumors to grow, rapidly and horrifically in some cases, ultimately causing seemingly unavoidable death—unless effective measures are taken in a timely fashion. Remember, cancer thrives on sugar.

You see, sugars serve as a super-charger for the insulin

hormone that actively promotes the growth of certain cells and particularly cancer. Heightening the danger even more to potentially critical levels, excessive "bad" sugars often accelerate the body's production of IGF-1, which normally is an internal biological product of the natural human growth hormone. Produced within the brain, particularly when sleeping while in the rapid-eye-movement (REM) state, human growth hormone is transported to the liver where it transforms into IGF-1. Within healthy children and young adults under normal, non-excessive conditions, IGF-1 is the major contributor to the body's natural and well-timed growth and strengthening.

Particularly until the mid-20s when the body's internal and natural HGH production steadily begins to decrease for the remainder of life, IGF-1 is vital and necessary for maintaining optimal health. Then, through the middle-age years and beyond, the steadily decreasing amounts of naturally produced IGF-1 are still needed, but only in sustainable and adequate amounts. (For more on this, see my popular books published in 2009, "Anti-Aging Cures," and "Your Secret to the Fountain of Youth, What They Don't Want you to Know about HGH Human Growth Hormone.")

Yet white sugar, particularly when eaten in excessive amounts, actually gives tumors what they desperately crave and need to grow and multiply. While also weakening immunity and thereby potentially leading to life-threatening internal inflammation, the sugars lead to a cascading effect that can eventually trigger the entire body's ultimate downfall.

Heavy People Get Cancer and Die

"Have you ever seen a super-fat person who is healthy at age 80 and beyond?" some cancer patients are occasionally asked.

"Although extreme exceptions occur, such people rarely exist. Before dying from cancer, heart problems or other organ failures, such individuals often spend their final months or even years in excruciating agony."

Everything comes down to the fact that eating excessive amounts of ice cream, gobbling down candy bars, and munching on carbohydrate-filled pizza makes the internal organs spin into destructive overdrive.

With cancer of the prostate, breast and other organs often the result, the liver gets forced into excessively high acceleration. This invariably creates a buildup of toxins, leading to eventual cancers while unsightly belly fat swells to unsightly and unhealthful levels.

For many of these people, the so-called "bad" foods might not seem so evident.

"I rarely eat sugary treats—and I avoid candy, cakes and ice cream," some of them might say. "I care about my health, and I take great care to monitor what I eat—so why is this happening to me? Why are my blood sugar levels excessively high? And, how did my belly get so big? Do you mean to tell me that this is why I've got cancer, or at the very least at this point that these factors put me in danger of getting the disease?"

Well, health professionals—particularly homeopaths that care about diet issues related to health—must give honest answers to such questions. While a specific cause of a particular patient's sugar-related ailments may never be known, the following seems true—at least based on extensive scientific research compiled in thousands of research reports: Cakes, candies, ice cream and treats are not the human body's sole source of simple sugars. Many people are unaware that the body transforms "refined carbohydrates" into simple sugars, using many brands of cereal, bread, pasta and even rice as sources for the destruction.

Positive News Emerges

Despite the "bad news" about sugar's destructive propensities, on the positive side homeopaths know that we can slow or entirely block the growth and spread of cancer and tumors by cutting off the body's supply of unhealthful, destructive sugars.

Cancer patients with high sugar levels have a lower survival time. Conversely, people with the disease who have low blood sugar live longer.

On a scientific and biological level everything comes down to the individual's "glycemic index." Sometimes called a "GI" this measurement lists the amount of glucose or "blood sugar" that the body has at a particular point in time.

For patients striving to control or prevent cancer, lose weight or manage diseases like diabetes, much of the effort hinges on regulating how fast and how long blood sugar levels rise. Within the realm of the Forsythe Anti-Cancer Diet this emerges into a critical factor. To achieve success or at least to get the best-possible results from their food-selection choices, patients must always remain fully cognizant of the fact that some foods push blood sugar levels up fast. As expected, many of the worst culprits are within the snack or "sugary treat" category like candy and ice cream. Yet until learning intricacies of this process, few people seem to realize that many common foods such as certain refined cereals, pasta and even white bread place high on the glycemic index. Such foods quickly transform glucose, elevating blood sugars—sometimes for prolonged periods.

High Index: Generally unhealthful foods considered high on the glycemic index also include corn flakes, white rice, pretzels, potatoes, and maltose—sometimes known as "malt sugar." You also should check food labels for maltodextrin, a moderately sweet and sometimes flavorless digestible food additive often used in soda and candy. All these foods are listed as high on the index, with the highest possible score a 100; all of them have an index listing greater than 70.

Low Index: Other foods get converted into glucose as well, but on a more gradual and healthier level, particularly those listed as low on the glycemic scale at listings of 55 or less, such as beans and some whole grains. The many foods within this range, some of them with antioxidant attributes listed earlier include: soy, black, pink, kidney and white beams from the legumes category; most types of fruits, especially mangoes, strawberries and peaches; sesame, pumpkin, poppy, flax and sunflower seeds; most types of vegetables, especially parsnip, beets and squash; many whole grains including barley, millet, oat, rye and brown rice.

Mid Index: Placed within the middle range of the glycemic index are a wide variety of foods that usually fail to place high on the list of recommended foods within the Forsythe Anti-Cancer Diet. These include bananas, which unlike most fruits that generally place low on the glycemic index contain a higher propensity to raise blood sugar. Other foods within this mid-range between 59 and 69 on the index are pita bread, prunes, raisins, grape juice, and regular ice cream.

Types of Sugars Vary

Thanks largely to the wide varieties provided by nature, the types of sugars vary in their sweetness and within vastly differing spectrums of the glycemic index. Some of the primary types of natural sugars within food are what scientists call "monosaccharide." Technically, these are the most important biological units within carbohydrates. Some sugars within the monosaccharide category taste sweet. Three of the most common, most frequently mentioned, each with its own unique potential impacts on blood sugar are:

Glucose: High on the glycemic index, and thus potentially the most dangerous of the three from an anti-cancer perspective, this also is sometimes called "dextrose" or "grape sugar." Cancer patients who see these words on a food label's list of ingredients should avoid buying or eating the product. Ironically, although glucose falls high within the glycemic index, according to numerous published reports scientists consider this sugar as a key or primary source of energy for the human body. In fact, despite its potential dangers as a sugar high on the glycemic index, according to numerous published reports it also serves as the brain's primary energy source. Food manufacturers derive glucose primarily from starchy crops, particularly rice, corn husk, wheat, sago, and maize. Cornstarch produced from maize is among glucose-containing foods high on the glycemic scale. Despite the potential dangers of excessive glucose consumption, seasoned and experienced homeopaths also explain that glucose is necessary for life.

Fructose: Sometimes called "fruit sugar," this is a basic monosaccharide found in most fruits. Because they're low on the glycemic scale, below the 59 level, and often feature a sweet taste, fructose sugars likely have a much lower potential than glucose for rapidly raising blood sugars. Fructose also has an extremely low danger of energizing tumors or cancer cells. Besides fruits, fructose is found in various other plants including flowers, berries, honey and the roots of some vegetables. Sugar cane, corn and sugar beets are among the most prevalent sources of fructose. Manufacturers sometimes combine glucose and fructose in making high-fructose corn syrup. Food producers often add fructose to drinks and foods to enhance flavor. Yet, "sneakily," at least from the perspective of some consumers, food manufacturers also reportedly use fructose as an additive to increase a particular product's "palatability." Rather than done just for enhancing flavor or taste, palatability is a process designed to make people who have previously eaten the specific foods to feel as if "deprived" after going without the meal for extended periods. When working as food producers hope, the subsequent re-eating of the meal triggers what experts call a "hedonic reward" within the brain. In terms that many lay people can easily understand, this means that a person "gets hooked" on a certain food—to the point where the individual psychologically feels as if he or she is addicted. For instance, do you have a difficult-to-break habit of eating high-sugar candy bars or the candies sold most frequently at movie theaters? Do you often fall back onto these foods, even after dieting as diligently and faithfully as you can for extended periods? Numerous scientists believe, at least according to some published reports, that the sense of palatability that food manufacturers strive to achieve depends on the same type of opioid-receptors within the brain that grips heroin addicts. If true, on a technical level this means that for people struggling to "get off junk food" while striving to control or prevent cancer, or to lose weight, kicking such habits might become as difficult as beating narcotics addictions.

Sucrose: Frequently called "table sugar," this falls within the middle range of the glycemic index. Deemed more harmful than the low-range, primarily fruit-based fructose sugars, sucrose also can pose potential dangers for cancer patients who are determined to prevent their tumors from receiving the energy that the disease yearns for and needs to grow. Besides being a major contributor to tooth decay, obesity, diabetes, gout and many other ailments, sucrose serves as the primary component in caramel candies—generated when this sugar decomposes at extremely high temperatures above 367 degrees Fahrenheit.

Some consumers insist that sucrose is unnatural, at least in the
highly dense bulk quantities at which it's distributed and eaten
today. On a worldwide scale sucrose was considered a luxury
before 1700, before rapidly achieving the rank of a "necessary"
food in the mid-1800s. Thus, like the tens of thousands of
variations of wheat today, does the human body lack the ability
to efficiently process, digest and absorb large or even small
amounts of sucrose in a healthful way? Or, as homeopaths believe,
does sucrose serve as an extremely unnatural and unhealthful
sugar, detrimental to overall public health? Well, the late widely
acclaimed U.S. physician Linus Pauling once proclaimed sugar
as the most dangerous food that Americans eat. Although vastly
diverse opinions exist on this throughout the worldwide medical
community, from everything I've seen homeopaths seem to
universally agree that sucrose poses extreme danger to the general
public. Boasting sweetness almost double that of glucose, sucrose
is the primary sweetener that cooks and food manufacturers use
in most of the "bad" snacks, cakes, candies or treats that seriously
endanger cancer patients and the overall public health.

Beware of Mercury

The processing of many sweet-tasting foods often involves
extremely dangerous mercury. Unlike the natural mercury
contamination of fish mentioned earlier, the food-manufacturing
industry actively processes sugar-laden foods and sometimes
even meals containing artificial sweeteners with this poisonous
substance. This intensifies white sugar's already-serious dangers.
Sadly, many consumers are never aware of mercury's impact,
and as a result the consequences could be disastrous. Besides
the potential of generating or contributing to cancer, the wide-
spectrum of horrible symptoms caused by mercury is life-

changing, debilitating or even fatal in the long-term. Built up over time, within children and adults, the excessive buildup of high mercury levels within the body creates many serious health problems. Besides the loss of teeth, hair and nails, persistent and sometimes life-long issues can include muscle weakness, profuse sweating, kidney dysfunction, memory loss, insomnia, rapid heartbeats, the dangerous shedding of skin, and a wide range of other serious problems too numerous to mention in full. Perhaps worst of all, from the perspective of cancer patients, elevated mercury could disrupt or slow the body's ability to generate essential white blood cells. Among the worst offenders:

High-fructose corn syrup: Used as a sweetener, this is produced when manufacturers process enzymes from corn syrups. This changes glucose—high on the glycemic scale and thus highly dangerous—into fructose, the much less dangerous sugar. However, consumers should refrain from getting fooled. Everything comes down to the fact that high-fructose corn syrup is an unnatural food found nowhere in nature. Throughout history until 1970 when manufacturing of this substance steadily accelerated, the human body never had to digest and process this dangerous substance. Multiplying the danger, the production involves caustic soda that scientists admittedly call "mercury grade." On a molecular level in terms that average people can easily understand, caustic soda has a highly caustic metallic base. Consumers need to know that "caustic" materials are actually corrosive substances that can literally destroy hard surfaces including metals and the surfaces of almost everything that high concentrations of this substance comes in contact with. The danger is so severe that in laboratory settings and even within everyday activities, people coming into contact with caustic substances can suffer extreme, life-altering damage to: the eyes, potentially a reduction of sight or blindness; the skin, with irreparable damage or intense scarring a possibility; severe respiratory damage; and severe and sometimes lifelong damage to the intestinal tract. Worsening matters, high-fructose corn syrup—rather than just mercury—has been blamed by some reports for causing obesity, non-alcoholic fatty liver disease and other ailments, all suspected potential precursors of cancer. Knowing this, would you eagerly and knowingly eat foods and drink beverages containing high-fructose corn syrup? Imagine the long-term effects on your body or those of your relatives, especially when they eat foods laden with this unnatural substance on a regular basis. Of course, working solely in their own best interest, food manufacturers will either tell the public that this material is "safe," or the corporations ignore the issue altogether. Once again, here we have a critical case where our corrupt or inept government, particularly the lame U.S. Food and Drug Administration, blatantly fails to work in the public's best interest. Instead of striving to protect the health of consumers, bureaucrats and politicians kowtow to high-paid food industry lobbyists that work solely to boost their employer's pursuit of the almighty dollar. Devilish and tricky, manufacturers might argue that this unnatural food is much cheaper than highly dangerous sucrose or common table sugar. Worsening matters on a broad scale, our federal government has the audacity to spend big bucks on subsidies to the U.S. corn industry to drive down the price of that crop—essentially feeding the hand that proverbially bites the American public. Shockingly, according to a 2010 report by the Economic Research Service, in 2008 the average American ate or drank a whopping 37.8 pounds of high-fructose corn syrup. Left on their own to protect themselves as best they can, consumers should avoid foods laden with this unnatural substance.

Soda pop: This food is perhaps the most dangerous.

According to a 1998 report by the Future of Freedom Foundation, in 1984 huge soda pop manufacturers including Coca-Cola and Pepsi began using high-fructose corn syrup for domestic production of their products—using that instead of cane sugar.

Soups: Within the overall public mindset, soup seems to garner a continuous reputation as generally healthy. Yet many consumers fail to realize that pre-made soups bought in cans often contain dangerous amounts of high-fructose corn syrup. People concerned about their weight or wanting to prevent or control cancer should always check soup labels, avoiding products that contain the unhealthful material. Wouldn't it be better to create your own homemade soup using natural ingredients?

Salad dressing: Instead of highly processed brands that show lots of additives and preservatives on labels, use natural products ranging from vinaigrette to extra-virgin olive oil. Lots of brands including some ranch dressings, depending on the manufacturer, contain natural substances including garlic, salt, herbs and spices that sometimes include mustard seed, black pepper and paprika.

Cereals: Look for "whole" or unprocessed brands, rather than selections jam-packed with additives like high-fructose corn syrup. At the same time, although a label might feature only what appears like natural ingredients, avoid refined products because those often feature dense, nutrition-deficient, high-sugar carbohydrates.

Packaged and Canned Food: Virtually all packaged and canned foods including frozen microwavable meals are potential targets for dangerous high-fructose corn syrup. So, take extra care to inspect labels.

Use Food-Selection and Lifestyle Strategies

While cognizant of the need to minimize unnecessary and potentially harmful sugars, anti-cancer advocates and consumers everywhere should make numerous relatively easy lifestyle changes. The first step involves a fasting glucose blood test to determine the amount of glucose in your blood. While the optimal range is usually considered between 70 and 90, health care professionals look for safe levels of the hemoglobin A1c. To get an accurate assessment of your overall long-term blood-sugar level, some doctors recommend getting similar tests about every three months. Ideally, patients must fast at least 12 hours immediately before technicians take their blood sample. If the tests indicate your fasting glucose is elevated a homeopath or dietitian can suggest foods likely to generate better results in subsequent tests. Even without a physician's direct advice, there are some steps consumers can take to lower glucose blood levels. Among them:

Protein: Eat protein-packed meals, since such foods can make you feel full or "satiated" for several hours while enabling blood sugars to stabilize to healthful levels. Some dietitians insist that breakfast remains each day's most important meal. So, eat plenty of high-protein foods as the day begins. Otherwise, you might essentially start the day off "on the wrong foot," unintentionally generating hunger throughout the day that can lead to excessive consumption of unnecessary sugars—particularly late into the night when the body is less likely to burn maximum calories.

Carbohydrates: These can skyrocket blood sugars, so at all meals—particularly during breakfast—avoid wheat-laden products like pastries, bread, bagels and pasta.

Balance: A critical strategy in managing or minimizing unnecessary sugars involves eating a balanced, varied diet. Instead of always eating only a handful of food types such as nuts and cheese, add adequate amounts of fruits, vegetables and non-red meats throughout the day—particularly antioxidant-rich foods.

Frequency: Make a concerted effort to eat regularly

scheduled small meals or light snacks every several hours throughout the day. This way when eating the right foods you'll give your body steady doses of the best sugars in ideal amounts that the body can easily and efficiently process. Going for extended periods of five or six hours of unnecessary fasting can lead to gorging excessively dangerous amounts of food and eating overly concentrated levels of sugar. Based on my observations over several decades, far too many people make the unwise and unhealthful decision of eating very little if anything throughout the bulk of the day. This often leads to extreme cravings, gobbling excessive high-sugar foods from the late afternoon well into the evening or even into the early-morning hours. Such lifestyles can lead to obesity and ultimately cancer. And, for people already with this disease, continuing such debilitating habits can and does often curtail the progress of their treatments or completely blocks health improvements. The excessive unnecessary sugars wreck everything.

Craving sweets: Humans have naturally craved sweets for thousands of years. So, to arbitrarily tell a person that "you never can have any sugary-tasting foods at all for the rest of your life" might seem like a pointless and even cruel strategy. There is good news for people who need or desperately crave at least some occasional speck of sweetness within their food. Without going overboard, most people can tolerate and enjoy lightly and naturally sweet foods. Generally healthy options include: stevia, a sweet-tasting herb; xylitol, a sugar alcohol about as sweet as sucrose but that actually helps dental health. Others include: maple syrup; agave, and raw honey. Most of these naturally sweet options contain nutrients, making them less capable than glucose and sucrose of pushing blood sugars to dangerous levels.

Artificial sweeteners: Why would any reasonable person

want to load his or her body with unnatural chemicals, even when striving to avoid dangerously high levels of natural sugars? Well, that's precisely what artificial sweeteners are, nothing but chemicals that endanger your health. So, in all instances avoid big-name brand artificial sweeteners even if they're advertised in print, radio and on TV as safe, viable and preferable sugar substitutes. Falling for this ruse can lead to various health problems, while continuing your cravings for sweetness and possibly generating toxic overloads that lead to cancer. So, avoid foods with labels featuring words like aspartame.

Hidden factors: Although some people feel great overall, they might be going about their everyday routines without ever realizing that their blood sugars are at dangerously high levels. As a result, potential or rapidly spreading sugar-related health problems can go fully undetected until health problems like cancer suddenly seem to become full-blown problems. Largely for this reason, besides actively working to minimize excessive sugar consumption, everyone should work to avoid becoming obese. You see, within people whose weight jumps above ideal levels, the body has an extremely difficult time efficiently processing sugars. Sadly, these combined factors sometimes ignite a rippling effect; as a person gets steadily heavier, the likelihood of gaining even more weight can and does become potentially greater over extended periods. Cancer sometimes results. Largely for these reasons—plus the hidden dangers of unseen high sugar levels, coupled with slow but steady weight gain—everyone should strive to maintain their "ideal weights." This holds true for people already overweight and for currently slim individuals, particularly young adults, who without even knowing this at the time, when continually eating unhealthful foods have a high probability of extensive weight gain over a period of several decades.

Body mass index: Often called "BMI" by health professionals, this is a measurement of whether an individual is overweight, underweight or maintains an ideal weight—based on the person's age, gender, height, and body type. If you're unsure if your weight is just right or too high, consider asking a health professional for a BMI status check. These charts do not actually measure percentages of body fat. In addition, for those unable to afford such checks or who lack the time or motivation, a simple naked-in-front-of-the-mirror review does the job just as well. A person who strips off all clothes and stands in front of a full-length mirror often gets an instant and clear vision of whether excess and unhealthful flab is a problem. Particularly if your results indicate overweight issues, you should immediately see a health professional such as a homeopath or a dietitian. As these experts help you develop a sensible diet, be sure to ask lots of questions about foods and lifestyle habits that can help properly manage blood sugar levels. In some instances, eliminating just one food from a person's lifestyle can help work wonders. For instance, three years ago one of my long-term patients, Wayne, eliminated his morning habit of ordering one large caramel iced coffee every morning at McDonald's. Just by making this single lifestyle change, coupled with the start of a regular continuous walking regime, Wayne lost 23 pounds that he has kept off. While still somewhat above his ideal BMI level, I recently gave Wayne detoxification integrative therapeutic supplements that helped remove toxins from his body. This, in turn, has been credited with indirectly helping Wayne benefit from a lowering of his lifelong sweets cravings.

Breast cancer: Excessive insulin or blood sugar production in the bodies of women often causes them to biologically resist excessive amounts of these substances. This hypersensitivity to elevated blood sugar levels likely helped generate their breast cancers. Certainly while all women can get this disease, both thin and heavy individuals, those who are overweight due primarily to excessively high sugar consumption will suffer the greatest risk of acquiring the disease. This is among the most urgent reasons why I strongly urge women who are overweight or obese to take immediate action to control their weight. These dangers come as a proverbial slap in the face to today's politically correct news media, which for the most part essentially tells all of society: "It's okay to be a heavy woman. They're regular people, too, and it's just fine if they spend the rest of their lives being overweight. That's their choice, which they have a right to make. Even heavy women have a right to appreciate and to be proud of their own physical beauty." Well, while careful to remain kind and level-headed, when responding to such statements I roundly proclaim: "Not so. What you're trying to force the general public to believe is nothing but political correctness." You see, by recklessly and foolishly clearing the way for such irresponsible statements, the news media and many publications are perhaps unwittingly creating an environment where heavy women eventually experience serious health problems. Besides heart disease, diabetes and an increased danger of stroke, sadly cancer sometimes emerges as a seemingly predictable outcome among overweight adult females. Thus, I choose to take a vibrant stand on this issue, telling any woman who might ask for my advice: "You need to take immediate action to control your weight issues, and sugar problems likely are a major cause of your obesity. To do otherwise is to invite heartache for yourself and for your family. Do you want your children to attend your funeral after you die at a relatively young age, or well before your prime or die when you're older? Odds seem strong that if you do not yet have significant health problems, as an overweight woman you almost

300

certainly will eventually experience them. And, simply telling the world that 'I've tried every weight loss technique imaginable and absolutely nothing works, so I eventually decided to accept myself for who I am,'—well, that's pure denial, and you've got to take more positive action now." Meantime, overweight men often carry similar issues throughout society, which from my personal view generally accepts them more than heavy women. Nevertheless, virtually everyone who is overweight today needs to take a more aggressive and determined role in achieving their ideal BMI level. Otherwise, we collectively could tell them: "Heart disease and very likely cancer are on their way to you. What have you done to prepare for your early demise? Have you already resigned yourself to death, and have you picked out your casket or burial plot yet?"

Chromium deficiency: Since the late 18th Century many scientists have suspected that people with insufficient levels of the vital metal chromium suffer from a severe inability to tolerate glucose. Since such sugars are necessary for life although high on the glycemic scale, people suffering from chromium deficiency sometimes experience confusion, severe or extensive weight loss, and impaired glucose tolerance. This problem has become so severe that an estimated 10 percent to 15 percent of U.S. adults may suffer from this condition, according to a 2004 report in "American Family Physician." If true, these statistics might point to a startling and continual upswing in the rates of cancers stemming from blood sugar level problems. In addition, numerous unverified, unsubstantiated reports claim that many people suffering from chromium deficiency could recover if they exercise, eat only healthy, controllable levels of adequate sugars, and lose from 5 percent to 7 percent of their body weight. Yet from my perspective as a homeopath, perhaps the best way to regain sufficient chromium levels is to eat only "whole foods," rather than processed foods.

Besides robbing foods of vital nutrients, the processing of these items often strips the essential trace elements. Once again, a critical health-related issue that could lead to cancer comes down to the fact that the vast majority of Americans lack any idea of what they're actually eating. Collectively as a society and individually, we all must do a much better job at watching, minimizing and ensuring our proper sugar intake—even if we're healthy, without cancer, diabetes or other diseases.

Chapter 29 Summary

People need to reduce their consumption of simple sugars or "white sugar" in order to minimize their chances of getting cancer, to refrain from becoming obese and to lose weight, and also to clear the bloodstream in order to improve the effectiveness of cancer treatments. Excessive consumption of white sugar often leads to obesity, a significant cause of cancer. Sugars are essential to life, and a wide variety of them occur naturally. Sugars high on the glycemic index are dangerous, potential carcinogens while those low on this measurement scale are generally safe. Sugars highest on the glycemic scale at 69 points and above are listed as "glucose," the most dangerous. In nature, glucose comes primarily from starchy crops like wheat, sago, maize, rice and cornhusk. Sugars listed as "fructose" below 59 on the glycemic scale are listed as the least harmful—but consumers should not be "tricked" because high-fructose corn syrup added to many foods is considered by some homeopaths as potentially carcinogenic. High-fructose corn syrup is used to strengthen the palatability of foods, making some consumers feel as if they're "hooked" on those dangerous meals. High-fructose corn syrup is hidden within many types of foods that are normally considered healthy, including soda pop, soups, cereals, salad dressings and packaged or canned meals. Within the middle range of the glycemic scale are "table sugars," packed into wide varieties of snacks that can cause numerous health problems—increasing the probability of getting cancer. Many consumers can cut down on unhealthful sugars merely by eliminating certain foods such as high-carbohydrate breads from their lifestyle habits. They also should avoid all types of artificial sweeteners, and strive to maintain their ideal weight on the "body mass index" or BMI scale. Many heavy women are in danger of getting cancer due to our politically correct attitudes that make these people think that "it's okay if I'm overweight." People also need to ingest adequate amounts of chromium, because studies show deficiencies in this metal may generate a severe inability to tolerate glucose.

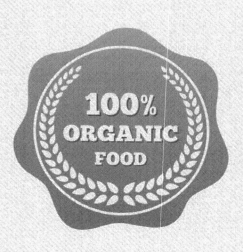

Chapter 30

Organic Foods

Those of us fully cognizant of the inherent dangers of processed foods, crops sprayed with chemicals and bio-engineered plants often eagerly seek "organic foods."

These supposedly are crops that have never been sprayed or pushed through mechanical processors. This understandably becomes a primary reason why everyone on a Forsythe Anti-Cancer Diet regimen strives to buy only organic produce. By limiting your meals to untainted natural selections, you'll minimize the amount of toxins that your body needs to process—potentially decreasing your probability of getting cancer. Also, this could minimize the loads of such invasive chemicals if you already have the disease.

But what precisely are "organic" foods, where can you find them and what information can you rely on to make such purchases? Although such queries might seem relatively simple, people learning about this issue often discover to their dismay that the various answers often emerge as confusing and perhaps frustrating.

You see, at least judging by what I've seen throughout the general news media and by scouring supermarkets, a huge number of foods are labeled as "natural" or "organic." Tragically, however, such labels do not always give the truth. Once again our government has failed us. Federal, state and local agencies often lack reliable and universal definitions on precisely what constitutes an organic food. Deceptive food distributors are able to use this loophole because technically virtually all plants and some farm animals are organic because they grow or are a part of nature.

Such skullduggery on the part of Big Food distributors in collusion with the lackluster Food and Drug Administration invariably tricks lots of consumers. The thought of these potential dangers boggles the mind. Just think of the number of people at this very moment who are eating tainted foods without knowing these dangers—wrongly thinking that they're doing the right thing by eating "organic."

Competition Compounds the Situation

Food chains that supposedly specialize in only natural or "whole" foods sprouted up faster than rampant weeds, picking up steam during the first decade of the 21st Century. Eager to protect themselves from pesticides, while hoping to achieve and maintain good health, hoards of eager consumers flocked to these new grocers. Some of those then-unique facilities at the time sold individual items at sharply inflated prices as compared to standard grocers.

Then, eager to seize upon steadily growing demand for organics, while fully aware that the new stores sold "natural" foods at relatively high prices, several giant department store chains eagerly entered the fray. Seemingly overnight for the first time many superstores that previously specialized and sold only non-food dry goods suddenly opened grocery departments, or added produce sections touted as "organic."

Complicating matters and determined to avoid losing a

substantial share of overall sales, the longtime standard grocers also began entering the fray. Seemingly just about every food sold in produce sections started getting labeled or touted as "organic." But are a number of those specific items actually sprayed or bio-engineered? Just as important, who from the government is actively and aggressively monitoring this situation on behalf of consumers? Well, coming as almost no surprise whatsoever to those of us aware of our government's incompetence, the answer is: "No one, at least on a strong, widespread and reliable scale."

Organics Spilled into Standard Food

The potential dangers imposed upon the general public intensified when the so-called "health food craze" spilled over from the produce sections to the regular aisles where canned, packaged and frozen microwavable foods are sold in standard grocery stores.

Once again, due largely to lax government oversight, food distributors that sell on a massive scale started embossing labels on highly dangerous, chemical-laden and potentially carcinogenic processed foods saying "natural," "organic," and "no trans-fats." Yet lots of these claims are deceptive. Although essentially labeled as good foods, lots of these products contain dangerously high levels of salts, sugars, trans fats, preservatives and pesticides.

Those of us determined to eat only natural, untainted and unmodified foods understandably become angered or frustrated by this. Just one of the major offenders here is a major peanut butter company with labeling that some consumers would consider deceptive, but only if they knew all the facts. Perhaps that particular situation stemmed from the startup of a much lesser known manufacturer of peanut butter, a brand sold solely in stores specializing in health food.

Well, that brand—called Product A here for descriptive purposes—is made solely from peanuts, with no preservatives, salt or added sugar. Then, after Product A started enjoying good overall sales thanks to its ability to meet high public demand, the huge longtime big-name peanut butter producer that historically had chemical-laden and sugar-laden products suddenly started making its own Product B—marketed with a huge label in large, bold-faced, deep-red letters: "Natural."

This was an obvious effort to remain competitive, tap into the organic food segment, or both. Deceptively, however, Product B contains intentionally added white sugars that can lead to obesity, cancer and other health issues. Worsening matters, although there are no apparent comprehensive studies to show this, does the added sugar increase the palatability of Product B—giving some consumers addictive-like cravings to it? Even more distressing, many consumers apparently fail to realize these possible dangers.

Increasing concerns multi-fold, the same or even worse potential problems could very well impact streams of other products labeled as "natural" or "healthy." Ultimately, the unwitting public overall gets victimized, targeted by giant corporations that collectively consider the bulk of society as "a bunch of stupid fools." Worsening the situation multi-fold, lots of public relations experts and lobbyists for these huge companies might actually start believing the corporations' misguided and deceptive propaganda—which some homeopaths prefer to describe as "hogwash."

Blame the News Media

Swallowing this gunk hook, line and sinker, the mainstream media sometimes falls for this ruse. Re-conveying the propaganda as "reliable fact," some TV talk show hosts and journalists sometimes spew this nonsense concocted by Big Food as if it were true.

As a key example, consider the nonsense that a Big Food representative rattled off during a chit-chat session during a major network morning talk show. Amid discussion on consumers eagerly hunting for organics, this person essentially said: "People don't realize this, but 98 percent of farms in America are family-owned. So, don't be fooled. There are more small farms out there than most people realize. The small, family-owned farms in the United States are not extinct or fading as many people wrongly believe. They're actually thriving."

Such verbal shenanigans failed to deceive those of us who carefully monitor the issue. You see, the lazy or incompetent talk show hosts either failed or refused to ask the tough questions that American consumers deserve. If the truth be told, a mere handful of major corporations grow, process and distribute the vast majority of foods sold in today's grocery stores. Meantime, the so-called 98-percent of family-owned farms combined collectively grow only an extremely small percentage of crops sold in the USA. This in turn should come as a shock or disturbing news at the very least to cancer patients and people striving to avoid the disease.

Imported Food Dangers

The overall potential dangers to public health are intensified even more, due to the fact that increasing percentages of foods sold today in American grocery stores are imported from other countries. At least the federal FDA in the USA has minimum guidelines capping the use of certain dangerous sprays. In many countries where food for American consumers is often grown, there are little or no national guidelines for farm-process safety or chemical limitations. Such blatant oversights were of less concern as recently as the 1960s, when the vast majority of foods sold in the United States were grown domestically—and immediately before the rapid increase in the processing of foods.

Today's consumers can cite several primary political, economic and scientific reasons for these changes detrimental to public health: food producers and distributors in other countries sought laborers eager to work for less money than that paid to migrant workers in the U.S.A.; rapidly spreading housing developments moved across former domestic farmlands, particularly in one of the breadbaskets of the world—Central California's San Joaquin Valley; improvements in the efficiency of the world's transportation infrastructure, enabling the shipping of foods in massive quantities—systems previously unavailable or once considered too expensive; and the acceptance of these foreign-grown foods by American consumers, most buyers fully unaware that these transitions seriously endanger their health.

These factors, individually and combined, open the doors to potentially deceptive practices overall within the food industry. With bogus labeling seemingly on the rise, American consumers often unknowingly find themselves endangered on a daily basis.

Due to no fault of their own, today's grocery store shoppers often lack any idea of where many crops on the shelves come from, whether they were sprayed with chemicals and how they were stored.

Combined and individually, these various negative developments leave me increasingly concerned for the long-term well being of my cancer patients, and for consumers everywhere who are simply trying what they think of as their best to maintain good health.

Food Shortages Endanger Health

Complicating matters for cancer patients and consumers

worldwide, severe international food shortages threaten to increase the likelihood that tainted foods will enter the marketplace. With steadily increasing intensity in recent years, economists and experts in the logistics of efficiently shipping crops have noted that food scarcity has critically endangered the health and pocketbooks of people from many societies. Economists and politicians blame the shortages on individual factors, or a combination of these issues including: extreme and dangerous weather seriously damaging or totally eliminating crops in specific regions—perhaps due to global climate change; attacks on crops by pests including insects or locusts, which sometimes multiply in horrific numbers due to adverse weather; hoarding by people eager to prepare for catastrophic food shortages; and stores that sharply rise prices of specific foods in efforts to gouge consumers, thereby potentially "causing a run on shelves" as people in specific neighborhoods or regions panic—rushing to buy food before it disappears from supermarkets.

A big question remains, specifically whether the chaos resulting from such tragic events increases the probability that tainted, cancer-causing foods or chemicals will reach the American marketplace.

Disturbing news that received scant attention in the mainstream American media in recent years chronicled "food riots," where people in other countries including Egypt essentially panicked. Rioters or looters broke into stores, shops and even residential homes. Many lawbreakers across widespread, diverse areas of Africa and Asia have looted for food.

While such violent events might not seem to have a direct impact on cancer-causing, food-based substances, perhaps Americans face a danger from food importers tempted to cram crops with preservatives. This way, perhaps, unscrupulous food producers and foreign farms strive to get their tainted crops to the United States—where such sellers are likely to get a higher price. The big losers here are multi-fold. First, consumers from third-world countries where the crops are grown face the possibility of severe food shortages or perhaps even starvation, particularly when their regions' critical harvests are shipped to the United States or elsewhere. And, secondly, any processed, tainted, high-sugar or chemical-laden foods from those countries would endanger the health of citizens of the USA, possibly increasing the likelihood of cancer.

Radiation Poses another Threat

As if the harsh worldwide economic conditions and the greediness of Big Food weren't already enough to cause grave concern, American consumers also face what some consumers describe as severe danger from radiation.

Lots of shoppers remain unaware that before reaching their store shelves crops including fruits and vegetables are intentionally exposed to radiation. This creates added concern among homeopaths because radiation in excessive amounts is a known carcinogen. As a typical American consumer you may have unknowingly purchased and consumed foods perceived as healthy, but in the process potentially exposed yourself to a much-feared cancer-causing substance.

The processors and importers of crops, who almost all insist that this food-preservation is safe, call the process as "irradiation." Such contamination sometimes rarely occurs in nature due to natural sources. But it's most often done intentionally by shippers and processors for what they boldly call the "sterilization of food."

To kill potentially harmful bacteria from massive quantities of food, particularly crops shipped in bulk, the major companies intentionally expose those crops to what these firm's call ionizing radiation in doses too small to cause significant danger to humans. But what happens to the bodies of people who eat huge quantities of irradiated foods at a single sitting, or who persistently ingest similarly tainted crops over extended periods.

While the impact of such dangers to people, and particularly to the potential impact of cancers, might seem inconclusive—with little doubt such processes pose significant possible public health threats. The various types of irradiation strategies include the exposure of food to gamma rays, X-rays and even electron beam processing.

Serious Health Implications

Besides killing bacteria, distributors also irradiate crops to halt or at least slow natural spoiling or degradation of the foods. Many consumers remain fully unaware that this has happened, sometimes within days or even hours before foods reach supermarket produce shelves. A wide variety of foods that seem to look normal or healthy to eat might be tainted this way, ranging from bananas and apples to asparagus.

"Holy cow!" some people exclaim when first learning these disturbing details. "This is almost the equivalent of standing in front of an operating X-ray machine for days on end. I'm concerned for myself and for my family."

Shockingly, parents who dearly love their children sometimes unknowingly expose the youngsters to the potential danger of irradiated foods. These people have every right to be angry.

On a molecular level, the irradiation process seeks to destroy the DNA of crops, creating enough internal damage that the foods lose the ability to repair themselves on a cellular level. Individual cells and ultimately the entire organism all die when exposed to radiation for extended periods. Well, this is much the same way that free radicals and cancer destroy the cells in living people, often obliterating vital DNA and eventually resulting in tumors and even death. Thus, the eating of irradiated foods becomes tantamount in some ways to exposing the body to the ravages of nuclear fallout or a nuclear explosion, as fully described in my 2011 book, the "Emergency Radiation Medical Handbook."

With this comparison in mind, think of the situation this way: "Would you eat crops or feed foods to your relatives, if those substances had been exposed to the ravages of a nuclear bomb or to the release of radiation due to an accident at a nuclear power plant?"

While some food industry advocates might argue that the irradiation process is carefully monitored and completely safe, the concerns among homeopaths intensify—especially when taking into account the fact that radiation is also used to increase the yield of juices, delaying crops from ripening and even to prevent certain harvests from sprouting.

On the positive side, at least according to a 1991 World Health Organization report, foods that undergo this treatment process do not become radioactive. Consumers also are being told to believe that after undergoing the procedure the foods do not spread radiation. Even so, should we believe everything that Big Food and politicians collectively tell us? Perhaps equally important, can major food producers be trusted, when they work en tandem with corrupt governments where politicians depend on campaign donations?

Certainly, irradiated foods are essentially being forced upon almost the entire world, whether or not consumers trust these companies and officials. According to a wide variety of news reports and articles, at least 59 countries allow irradiation. Regulations vary greatly despite the widespread acceptance of this potentially dangerous procedure. Some nations specify that only specific crops can undergo irradiation, while other countries permit every type of food.

Labeling of Irradiated Foods

Par for the course, within the USA the Food and Drug Administration drops the proverbial ball once again on this critical issue. The FDA requires a Rodura symbol on only some foods that have been irradiated. Unaware what the symbol means, consumers might mistake the logo as the symbol of a food manufacturer, or even some sort of signal that the product is healthful or natural. The symbol is a green circle, embossed at the center with another green round dot surrounded by white. Underneath the green dot spreading to both sides from the center rests leaf-like symbols. In essence, the human eye is lead to believe that everything is natural, when in fact quite the opposite is true.

Worsening matters, the required labeling is only done on what some well-informed consumers might call a "hit-and-miss" basis. Federal regulations also require explicit language describing conditions where the food can be used, or describing how the food was changed.

While on the surface such efforts might sound admirable, ask yourself or other people if they have ever seen such labels and if they know that the language means. Invariably, you probably will find, the answer is a resounding "no," coming to the conclusion that a vast majority of people have absolutely no idea of the issue.

Topping this off, within the United States restaurants have absolutely no requirement to label meals as containing irradiated foods, or to tell consumers about the issue.

The Potential for Cancer Emerges

Thanks to the hard, diligent and efficient work of various

consumer rights organizations, many people have been able to express worries of what they describe as potentially serious side effects from irradiation. While the need for study and comprehensive research on this issue remains high, some health experts have become increasingly concerned about cancer dangers. Among just a handful of the potential adverse reactions feared by consumers:

Bacteria: Besides performing the jobs for which it was intended, irradiation kills so-called "good" bacteria that otherwise would help urgent and necessary processes within the digestive system. As studies previously mentioned clearly indicate, serious disruption of the intestinal tract's processes can block the absorption of vital nutrients—gradually setting the stage for potential toxic overload, and ultimately cancer. Meantime, some consumers worry that irradiation sometimes encourages the growth of bacteria that's deemed "bad." Under worst-case scenarios, the combined conditions of eliminating "good" while promoting "bad" could clear the way for severe damage to the digestive tract.

Toxins: Various consumer watchdogs also reportedly claim that irradiation sometimes fails to destroy bacterial toxins. As we've already seen, such substances can damage the liver, destroying the healthful processing of bile and thereby creating a potential factory for cancer.

Top Recommendations

Even in the wake of these genuine concerns, however, ultimately as far as I can tell there has never been any conclusive, irrefutable evidence of any direct link between food irradiation and cancer. Nevertheless, due primarily to the multiple and simultaneous potentials for extreme cancer-related dangers, I strongly advise consumers to:

Labels: Check all labels for the FDA Rodura symbol, or for written descriptions, and avoid such foods in all instances.

Communications: Without trying to seem alarmist, casually tell your friends and family how and why they should avoid irradiated food.

Professional: Ask your doctor, homeopath or dietitian for specific advice on whether to avoid such foods, particularly while recovering from illnesses including cancer.

Restaurants: If the business offers the types of food most likely to be irradiated, ask your server if the meals underwent that process. According to the U.S. Department of Agriculture, the most prevalent irradiated foods sold domestically are ground meat products, dried spices, spinach and tropical fruits grown in diverse locations ranging from Florida and Hawaii to India.

Other Primary Organic Food Issues

Some scientists and economists claim that organic pesticides comprised of natural substances generate just as much environmental damage as manmade chemicals used for similar purposes. Sharply disputing these claims, proponents insist that overall, organic farms offer greater diversity than giant conventional plant-growing facilities, conserving more energy and costing less than Big Food.

Heightening these arguments, the money-hungry allies of gargantuan conventional farming insist their facilities are far more economical and beneficial to society. These agencies, firms and lobbyists claim Big Food generates far more crops per acre, ultimately minimizing costs for consumers, distributors and sellers.

No matter who "wins" these arguments, usually behind the scenes with scant news media attention, the potential big loser becomes the health and safety of the general public. Left to their own devices and struggling as best they can to go about their everyday lives, average people have little time or money to enter this political fray.

Despite these formidable hurdles, consumers everywhere should still do their utmost to ensure that they and their families consume only natural "organic food."

Yet while continually aware that we're virtually surrounded with unhealthful, processed or non-organic food wherever we go, how many of those meals should be considered as too much? Well, from the view of many homeopaths and seasoned dietitians, you should never eat such selections—not even once. This strategy alone might seem ridiculous and downright impossible to many people. After all, even seasoned practitioners of medicine need to acknowledge that there apparently have been no seasoned, in-depth studies into whether eating a single meal containing sugar-laden, processed and chemical-filled foods would cause cancer or other serious health issues.

Even so, many seasoned practitioners of natural medicine might argue that having one caramel-covered, sugary candy bar every Sunday could gradually cause extensive health damage over time. You see, the human body certainly "works wonders," generating miracles designed for its own self-preservation on a continuous basis—fighting invaders and creating new cells.

But essentially loading small but regularly ingested meals of harmful foods into the body could very well be even worse in the long run than the ravages caused by a low-dose chemotherapy regimen over a similar time span. You see, although "bad" foods are essentially low-grade poisons, chemically in a much different way than chemo drugs, such meals serve their wretched purpose in endangering or damaging the body.

Any mother with basic intelligence and common sense would

never want to intravenously pump chemo drugs every Sunday into her children if they've never suffered from cancer. With just as much urgency, the same parent should be forcefully avoiding and prohibiting their children from eating high-sugar, highly tainted foods every Sunday, or on any day for that matter. Even so, angered by such strategies, many adults might argue that candy, ice cream bars and sugary treats have been enjoyed by families and especially children for many generations with no apparent serious health problems.

Try Using Common Sense

While no specific studies have been done over multiple decades of specific individuals involving this issue, there can be no denying that cancer and obesity rates among children and adults have steadily increased in the United States.

Perhaps much of this suffering involves people who wrongly think that "I have been eating well. How in the world did this happen to me?"

With little doubt the average American seems to lack any notion that most foods, especially pre-packaged meals or snacks sold at typical grocery stores may pose serious cancer threats. Eating these unhealthful items on even a sporadic, intermittent basis could easily become a long-term recipe for disaster. Although many practitioners of standard medicine might sharply disagree, how can they explain booming cancer and obesity rates among adults and children?

Surely pushing caramel from the top of the glycemic scale into the digestive system just once per week threatens the liver, gallbladder, bile system and digestive tract—while generating an overload of protective white blood cells and also increasing the long- and short-term dangers of free radicals.

By comparison, many mechanics, hooligans and vandals

know that by sticking just one cup of sugar into an automobile's gasoline tank they can permanently damage or even destroy the engine. Practitioners of natural medicine consider the human body just as sensitive to outside invaders. This becomes critical when considering the fact that built up over time the consumption of just one sugary candy bar every week is the equivalent of several pounds of pure cancer-causing, obesity-causing white sugar collectively over an entire year.

By the time cancer is discovered and the person sees an oncologist for the first time, whatever created the disease is invariably not among top issues to address. By then, from the view of standard doctors, it's "too late to turn back now, too late to worry about any causes. Instead, we need to address your health issue by giving you poison—chemo."

Knowing this potential outcome beforehand, the advice homeopaths would give is, "Take decisive action now to avoid non-organic foods. Avoid putting yourself into a position where you will ever need to hear such 'you've-got-cancer' statements, and then find yourself struggling to remain alive."

Pathetic Government Labeling Strategies

Finally bowing to heated complaints from numerous consumer organizations, the U.S. Congress passed the Organic Food Protection Act of 1990. Besides administering a label designating foods that supposedly are certifiably "organic," the legislation also formed a division within the U.S. Department of Agriculture to enforce and administer these regulations. A typically cumbersome and overly bureaucratic agency, in 1990 the USDA finally posted its rules in the Federal Register.

Dubbed the National Organic Program, often called the "NOP," this agency monitors and regulates every phase that eventually impacts consumers—production, processing and sales. This system is supposed to stipulate how a food producer, processor and seller earns the right to label a specific food as "organic."

Yet sadly, probably because bureaucrats are involved and since Big Food got its proverbial greasy hands into this realm, only 95 percent of a specific food needs to contain "organic" ingredients in order for that product to qualify for the USDA Organic Seal.

Is this devilish, or do our nation's bureaucrats think consumers are naïve—or both? Since up to 5 percent of a product can contain non-organic materials and still get such a seal, what are those potentially dangerous substances? Consumers and natural health advocates certainly have a right to show concern, especially since not all ingredients are necessarily listed. Compounding the problem, even according to the USDA's own estimation, a mind-boggling 56 separate public agencies collectively work to oversee domestic certification of foods within the United States.

At least according to some reports, the National Organic Program directly employed only 30 people in 2010. Imagine that, the equivalent of a classroom filled with individuals managers collectively oversee the compliance of the entire gargantuan multi-billion-dollar organic industry. Could such relatively small staffing levels lead to a lack of proper oversight? Are there cases where products embossed with the Certified Organic seal actually contain more than 5 percent of chemicals, preservatives and unnaturally refined foodstuffs?

Fast-Paced Society Complicates Matters

As far back as the late 1940s when limited numbers of consumers launched what sociologists call the early "Green Revolution" for organic foods, these advocates urged each other to "know your farmer." For the next few decades personal, direct communications with farmers were deemed the only way to determine if that person sprayed crops with potentially harmful chemicals.

Taking this direct-contact strategy into today's complex business and government infrastructure, anyone advocating such a strategy might proclaim: "Know your bureaucrat, plus who that person has interacted with, how and why." Since such efforts obviously would be fruitless, the challenges for today's consumers increase multi-fold. Exacerbating this problem, the operators and owners of small farms are disappearing at least in terms of their overall impact on nationwide food consumption on a percentage basis.

Controversy Continues

These controversies continue to erupt although a huge variety of studies have been unable to find any differences between the impacts on human health, generated by organic foods and by tainted, processed, chemical-laden Big Food crops. Allies of these giant industries insist that researchers have yet to find conclusive scientific evidence that conventional foods are less safe or healthful than organics.

Even so, many consumers insist the potential contaminations include feeding tainted or inadvisable foods to cows, and keeping tens of thousands of animals like chickens or turkeys cooped up together in tight spaces. People concerned with what they call "health threats" from these processes insist that animals be "roaming;" these consumers prefer packaging that gives this designation—including eggs from chickens that aren't crammed together in tight cages throughout their short, miserable lives.

According to statements issued by the Obama administration in September 2012, the fastest growing food sector at the time in the USA was organics. If true, this shows that overall consumers were getting wise to the pernicious tactics of Big Food, sharply pushing up demand for untainted crops.

From the perspective of a homeopath and as an oncologist, all these varying issues come down to a single factor—cancer. At least in public forums, few people would openly argue against giving consumers the right to protect their own health and that of their families. But two sharply conflicting issues come to play, potentially putting the lives of many people at risk. The differing perspectives stem from vastly diverging goals. On one hand we have everyday people struggling financially, often choosing highly dangerous, quickly packaged and often sugar-filled meals loaded with excessive carbohydrates. The only foods they can afford are mass-produced, chemical-filled and sugar-laden, high-carbohydrate meals. These individuals seem to comprise the general masses that Big Food is trying to serve, using harmful technologies to produce as much food as quickly and as simultaneously as possible—in order to get crops efficiently and cheaply to the market. All along, numerous people with the time, knowledge and financial resources decide to buy their groceries at organic food supermarkets, where many observers insist the items cost much more than at regular stores. Herein, various formidable and life-impacting questions arise, primarily: "Are we in a situation where only upper middle-class and wealthy people can afford untainted and natural organic foods, while the poor or the uneducated feel they have no other option than to buy relatively inexpensive, unhealthy foods?"

All these various issues are so highly complex and intermingled, making any answers would seem incomplete as huge segments of society face these critical issues head-on. Particularly among cancer patients and people striving to avoid the disease, here are vital challenges and issues to consider—plus possible solutions in some instances:

Costs: If you're a consumer on an extremely limited budget, what can and should you do to buy the healthier foods? This challenge could emerge as formidable, seemingly impossible to overcome in some instances. Food banks designed to help the needy nationwide are crammed with highly dangerous foods, unhealthy cereals, sugar-laden snacks and highly processed meats. Much of the time, these foods are given to families that have nothing else to eat. Faced with no other options, and perhaps often unaware of the dangers, poor or jobless parents bring these foods home to their families. As a result, it should be no surprise that obesity and cancer rates seem to be rising steadily in low-income regions across America. Due to no fault of their own, obese poor people live in diverse communities nationwide. Unemployed or with insufficient incomes, streams of these consumers rely on food stamps—which they use at standard supermarkets that lack sufficient supplies of organic foods. Invariably many of these consumers buy mostly tainted, processed, sugary groceries, while struggling just to make ends meet from month-to-month. To these individuals, caring and knowledgeable homeopaths and other practitioners of natural medicine likely would recommend: "Just do the best you can. Find and buy the most organic options within the store that you can afford. And, have you ever thought of growing your own crops at home? Most seeds are relatively inexpensive, especially low when compared to the cost of buying the specific food items at their maturity off supermarket shelves." Meantime, to the more affluent consumers who often go to organic food stores or to regular supermarkets that offer such selections, the advice would be: "Check the labels, and ask lots of questions of the store's personnel." Interestingly, even at organic food stores non-scientific, informal surveys of the regular grocery aisles outside the produce sections often reveals streams of packaged foods—some loaded with excessive salt, sugars and even preservatives. So, ultimately, no matter what their backgrounds, education levels, wealth or social status, essentially "all of us are in this dangerous situation together, and each of us needs to do the very best that we can to understand, adjust to and cope with these issues."

Availability: Some consumers live in isolated rural desert or mostly uninhabitable areas where growing their own foods would become challenging. Many of these people and others on limited incomes from highly populated urban areas often find themselves with little or no choice other than to buy their groceries from stores supplied only by Big Food. These individuals can "grin and bear it," or make the aggressive, continuous effort to spend the time and resources to either grow as much of their own food as they can. Taking a concerted effort to briefly venture outside of a particular neighborhood or community simply for the purpose of buying preferred organic foods takes gumption, commitment and stick-to-itiveness. Such efforts can emerge as cumbersome, seeming downright impossible, particularly in today's fast-paced society where just about everyone seems pressed for time and for money in a depressed economy. To these individuals, some homeopaths might suggest: "What about getting your organic food through the mail? Is that an expense you're capable of and willing to take? And, how about in-person, front-door food delivery services operated by local companies or by satellite distributors of natural foods? Growing numbers of such services can often be found online, and steadily increasing numbers of consumers are posting their online personal reviews of such services. By opening up your mind to the positive possibilities of technology, if you can afford to, perhaps you'll be able to make such food-ordering routines a positive and healthy lifestyle habit."

Consistency: Any efforts to buy only organic foods or to grow crops at home can only be effective when done on a consistent, unbending and reliable way on a long-term basis. Merely doing these things for brief periods—or just for a few years before stopping them—will not enable consumers to reach their long-term goals. Remember, the objective should be to live a lengthy, healthy, and relatively stress free life until an extremely old age—eventually dying in your sleep without having to endure the terrible physical pain of cancer, or having to withstand rigorous chemotherapy. To receive any positive long-term impact, you should make this lifestyle more than just a mere preference. Striving for good health, and eating healthful foods needs to become a permanent habit, an unbendable mindset—even for those who already have cancer. As we've seen from the integral discussion so far, we live in a highly complex society where the dangers and challenges seem to be increasing every day. Based on reliable findings by scientists, there should be no reason for emotional shock and denial whenever we hear that someone has just been diagnosed with cancer. Ultimately all you can personally do is simply "the best that you can"—particularly eating or preparing only natural, untainted food—to minimize the probability that you, a family member or a loving companion will get this disease.

Role model: There's little to gain from lecturing your children or relatives on the importance of a healthy anti-cancer diet, unless you're "walking the walk." Parents of young children need to realize that their offspring's formative years will soon seem to have passed in a flash. So, simply imposing stringent "no-candy" rules and "no-cola" restrictions will not do anywhere near enough to help ensure that they carry on such admirable intentions, eventually making their own good-food lifestyle choices upon reaching adulthood. A logical, productive and highly effective way to make this happen in the long-term is to bring them to the grocery store with you. Start from their earliest years, before continuing clear through their teens. Every step of the way, you should never buy "junk food." Gradually as they grow older have your children assist in making the food selections. Eventually as your youngsters gain more responsibility in their late teens, send them to the grocery store with the plan of returning with only healthy food. Along the way, either you or your children might get off track in such a lifestyle, since as the old saying goes "to err is only human." Nonetheless, especially if you want your children to eventually grow up with the best chance for long, relatively healthy lives, you can help put these positive motions into full gear early. The same strategy should hold true for parents who are just beginning to embrace a good-food lifestyle, at a point when their children are teens or already adults. Imagine their reaction when they observe such positive change in you. That alone could go a long way toward motivating them to launch anti-cancer diets of their own. Additional opportunities sometimes emerge when adults eventually discover that their aging parents suffer from cancer. Rather than dwelling only on the negatives, such instances also can present opportunities to help your loved ones. While assisting their mature parents in adopting their own health food lifestyles, routines and preferences, adult children often get to discover the joys of healthy foods for the first time. Like I sometimes tell patients, "It's never too late to discover just how fun, tasty and healthful that organic foods can be for us all."

Chapter 30 Summary
People everywhere should strive to eat primarily "organic" foods that have not been sprayed, packed with chemicals, quickly

packaged or bio-engineered. To do otherwise could expose you to the extreme dangers of known carcinogens. Always be aware that some Big Food companies strive to "trick" consumers into buying and eating foods that are not actually organic. In some instances, foods touted or advertised as natural actually have been packed with cancer-causing white sugars. Always remaining fully aware that Big Food considers many consumers as "fools," be sure to check labels of all food products for ingredients even on meals listed as supposedly natural or organic. Some potential carcinogenic dangers come from imported, improperly labeled crops. International food shortages, particularly during major disasters like hurricanes, increase the dangers as manufacturers rush to prepare and ship crops to the United States. Compounding these problems, Big Food also sometimes blasts crops with radiation as a preservative measure while these foods are en route to American grocery stores. Some medical professionals fear this may pose potential risks, although such danger has never been scientifically proven. Some consumer organizations fear this irradiation process could harm or kill "good" bacteria that would otherwise help the intestines. Ineffective labeling requirements overseen by the inept and corrupt U.S. Food and Drug Administration has done little to help the public on this vital issue, while packaging labels remaining confusing to many consumers. Everyone interested in benefiting from the Forsythe Anti-Cancer Diet regimen should carefully follow ongoing developments on this issue. All along, poor or mostly uneducated people may continue to eat primarily dangerous, cheap, processed foods, possibly because most of these consumers remain unaware of the issue or they lack funds to purchase or locate organic crops.

Chapter 31

Acid vs.
Alkaline

As briefly mentioned earlier, cancer usually loves and flourishes an in acidic environment. The opposite occurs when cancer is exposed to highly alkaline substances. These factors warrant significant discussion due primarily to probability of using these attributes to prevent or destroy the disease. Many of us learned in high school chemistry class that acid and alkaline are on a measurement scale that scientists call "pH," the listing of a substance's hydrogen ion concentration. Pure water rests at the middle of the pH scale with a ranking of number 7 when at 25 degrees Celsius.

Organisms and chemicals below 7 on the pH scale are within the acidic range with the strength or degree of acidity increasing toward zero. The opposite is true for alkaline, anything from above 7 to the maximum 14.

A comprehensive listing of the acidity and alkalinity within specific foods is so voluminous that showing them in full would fill the size of a large dictionary. Yet for basic explanatory purposes, here are some of the primary foods within each category:

Acidic foods: Remember, these generally are foods that you should avoid or eat only in minimum quantities because cancer thrives in acid environments. Perhaps one of the most dangerous is soda pop, because phosphoric acid is a primary component of such beverages, which cancers also love due to high sugars or artificial sweeteners. Laboratory researchers have found evidence that phosphoric acid decreases or minimizes essential bone density, while also possibly endangering the kidneys. Damage to these organs and the bones might generate overall bodily defects, setting the stage for potential cancer. Some foods, especially certain specific varieties of citrus fruits might—paradoxically —also serve as excellent antioxidants. Unripe mangoes and tamarind contain natural tartaric acid. It also occurs naturally in many other plants including bananas and even grapes. Various other citrus fruits including lemons and oranges have citric acid. This poses potential concern for cancer patients, because citric acid in concentrated form is so corrosive that it's often used in cleaning products. Compounding the potential confusion for consumers, other foods often touted as super-healthful contain varying amounts of oxalic acid, particularly rhubarb and the carambola fruit—sometimes called "starfruit," plus spinach and tomatoes. The dangers of excessive acids are so severe on rare occasions within nature that these substances can reach poisonous levels. Consumers and especially people who grow their own crops at home should avoid the leaves of rhubarb and carambola, which contain highly toxic levels of oxalic acid. In fact, many people fail to know this, but a huge variety of seemingly healthy foods eaten regularly by consumers also contain potentially dangerous oxalic acid. Yet thankfully, in the vast majority of those crops, the levels of oxalic acid are miniscule. Although in-depth, intensive and long-term studies apparently still need to be done on this potential issue,

330

the possible dangers of these oxalic acid-containing foods seem extremely minimal or non-existent. Nonetheless, some homeopaths might choose to recommend the following foods be eaten only intermittently as regular-size servings—and never in bulk, massive quantities as your only source of food. With generally miniscule oxalic acid content, they include: cabbage, asparagus, broccoli, carrots, eggplant, squash, turnips, sweet potatoes and watercress. According to a 2005 research report from Oxford University, the lowest-published lethal dose of oral oxalic acid is 600 mg/kg—causing fatal kidney failure because it causes calcium oxalate, the major component in kidney stones. While these factors generate obvious reasons for concern, some foods generate certain acids that serve as essential biological components of elements necessary for human life. This is especially true for Vitamin C, also called "ascorbic acid," derived from citrus fruits including oranges, plus guava and lemons. Remember, as stated earlier, a lack of Vitamin C in people causes scurvy, which generates a host of serious health issues including a loss of teeth or even death. Our bodies also naturally and internally produce various biological acids necessary for life. Key among these is lactic acid, sometimes called "milk acid," generated by muscle activity. This process serves as part of the normal metabolisms in people, many animals and some plants. Within humans, lactic acid is generated by our normal metabolisms and even exercise. A variety of other bodily fluids and organ systems also contain natural but necessary acids, including the blood, pancreas and skin—with some levels actually above 7 on the pH scale, the range usually occupied primarily by alkaline. But the highest, most acidic internally produced acid by far is gastric acid—which comes in at a whopping number 1, the highest range of acidity. A digestive fluid formed by cells in the stomach's lining, gastric acid serves a critical role in the digestion process. This brings up an interesting and logical question: "Because cancer thrives and yearns for an acidic environment within the human body, why don't all people get the disease— since we eat acid-containing foods that are usually good for us, and because our bodies internally generate natural acids?" Well, while intricate books and scientific papers could emerge from this issue, everything essentially comes down to the fact that when healthy our bodies regulate acids, keeping them at manageable levels that are unlikely to cause cancer. But this amazing natural counter-balancing gets kicked off-kilter when excessive amounts of acids get formed—sometimes as a result of excessive or unhealthful sugars or other unhealthful substances. For instance, the excessive buildup of plaque in our mouths can generate a highly localized acidic environment, potentially resulting in tooth decay.

Alkaline foods: For the most part cancers often dislike, fail to thrive in or even die or become dormant within highly alkaline environments—the complete opposite of what often occurs in excessive levels of acidity. Largely for this reasons, many homeopaths seek to recommend foods leaning more toward the alkaline range higher up on the pH scale. These health professionals and dietitians often refer to this strategy as an "alkaline diet." Proponents of this strategy believe that certain foods, particularly those high on the alkaline range, positively impact the acidity of body fluids.

A primary goal becomes lowering the acidity of our urine and blood. Many practitioners of alternative medicine believe alkaline diets sharply decrease the probability of cancer, while also potentially assisting overall health amid treatments for those with the disease.

Ideally, this overall strategy works best when specifically

chosen, alkaline-heavy foods help in the effective regulation of what scientists call "acid-base homeostasis." In terms that an average person might better understand, this means creating an ideal balance between the natural acids within our bodies and the ideal "base" or preferred good-health balance among various specific atomic structures within the body.

On a chemical level, a "base" has molecular or atomic properties that are the opposite of acids. Technically, bases reduce the concentrations of hydronium ions within water, while acids do the opposite. Within the realm of acid-base homeostasis, serious unbalanced situations can occur. Too much base in the blood causes alkalosis or "alkalemia," causing many negative symptoms including muscular weakness.

Another ailment, "acidemia," or acidosis, stems from elevated acid levels in the blood—sometimes generating respiratory ailments, including chronic illnesses. Diseases potentially impacted by or related to acidosis reportedly sometimes include muscular dystrophy and late stages of emphysema. While these and many other potential diseases often associated with acidosis generate concern, cancer is one of the most predominant afflictions that natural health practitioners seek to prevent or minimize with alkaline diets.

Alkaline Diet Issues

Some researchers also worry that despite the potential anti-cancer benefits of alkaline diets, they simultaneously believe that too much consumption of meals consisting of primarily alkaline-rich foods may increase the risks of osteoporosis. Even among medical professionals, some argue that such theories aren't backed up by reliable medical research.

Similar claims also erupt regarding the overall supposed

effectiveness of alkaline diets. For these reasons, coupled with
the apparent possible osteoporosis danger, consumers should only
attempt such food regimens under the care, advice and monitoring
of a medical professional. Generally, although specific strategies
might seem to vary, overall, these food regimens strive to avoid
cheese, grains, meat and poultry.

Some practitioners of natural medicine insist that testing
in the 1800s by French biologist Claude Bernard indicated that
carnivorous diets focused primarily on meat increase the body's
acidity—a condition that many researchers subsequently blamed
for encouraging the growth and spread of cancer. Conversely,
according to results from Bernard's research, herbivore diets
consisting primarily of plants increased the body's overall alkaline
levels—conditions that today's researchers say discourages the
formation, growth and spread of cancer.

If true, at least according to various 20th Century research
projects, foods high in sulfates, chloride and phosphates increased
acid levels. Diets containing magnesium, potassium and calcium
were found to increase alkalinity. Complicating matters, some
alkaline-laden foods including plums, cranberries and prunes
actually increased hippuric acid levels in urine, according to studies
first reported in 1985.

Diverse Issues Remain

Overall, despite the paradoxical results of some tests,
according to a 2009 dietitian journal, foods that frequently produce
acids are eggs, meat, fish, poultry and cheese. Such results might
confuse anti-cancer diet advocates, since eggs and some fish
species possess antioxidant or attributes that discourage free
radicals.

Vegetables and some fruits increase alkaline levels,

particularly those that don't contain citrus acids, like cranberries and prunes. Technically, the "alkaline ash" and "acid ash" generated by the combustion of these is what the body absorbs, not necessarily the acids that were in these meals before they were eaten. Thus, although scientists generally consider citrus fruits as acidic, the same researchers often insist that such crops are considered "alkaline producing;" the fruits generate alkaline ash rather than acid ash when combusted.

The Canadian Cancer Society entered the fray in August 2012, essentially stating in summary that there has been no scientific evidence to back up the claims of some alternative medicine practitioners that alkaline diets are effective in treating cancer.

Targeting the lay audience, various homeopaths insist that besides treating cancer, other potential benefits include using this diet for heart problems, weight loss and low energy. To varying degrees and differing levels of overall public exposure, these numerous positive claims by alternative medicine practitioners have been chronicled in books, magazines and on Websites plus direct-mail advertisements.

Backed by Big Pharma and Big Food, the mainstream media might be playing an excessive role in striving to shoot down the believability of such positive claims. After all, those giant industries have a lot to lose financially if more consumers start avoiding processed foods and pharmaceuticals—which some versions of the alkaline diet strongly recommend avoiding.

Huge food and drug corporations spew out bogus propaganda, striving to serve their own best interests rather than taking the best course of action for consumers and for patients. Overall these deceptive "misinformation campaigns" strive to portray alternative medicine practitioners as "quacks" who try to push whacky treatments upon an unsuspecting public.

Mindful of these deceptive tactics, consumers need to know that homeopaths as an overall segment of the medical industry are highly professional. Just as important, highly educated practitioners of natural medicine have just as much or even more education and training than standard allopathic physicians.

To strive to discount the potential benefits of alkaline diets and to put the professionalism of those who recommend them into question is tantamount to an extreme fraud on the general public. As already shown here the many potential positive impacts of alternative medicines—particularly healthful foods—are based largely on sound, reliable and consistent scientific research.

Understand the Issue

With these overall factors and issues clearly understood, as one of only a handful of integrative medical oncologists in the United States—with extensive experience in both standard and alternative medicines—I strongly proclaim, without any reservation whatsoever, that healthy, alkaline-inducing foods can go a long way in the battle against cancer. Homeopaths should continue to play an integral role in discouraging patients from allowing allopathic physicians to order these people to rely solely on dangerous drugs while avoiding natural foods as viable factors within overall treatment.

Knowing this, along with the thousands of homeopaths nationwide, I have a responsibility to tell you the truth about the potential benefits of high alkaline foods—plus low-sugar antioxidant crops that are likely to individually and collectively help improve and strengthen health.

"Shame on the prognosticators—those who would strive to discourage or to prohibit even a consideration of a sensible alkaline diet," I tell some patients. "By all means, make no hesitation in seeking the professional advice of homeopaths and experienced dietitians on this critical issue."

Major Organizations Join the Fray

Often supported by Big Pharma, standard oncologists and the inept Food and Drug Administration, some major non-profit health organizations and federal agencies recklessly claim that the supposed benefits of alkaline diets and of alternative medicines are nothing but "myth." Shockingly, in just one incidence of such tomfoolery, in August 2012 the American Institute for Cancer Research issued a statement insisting that any claim that the alkaline diet can significantly change blood processes is "contrary to everything we know about the chemistry of the human body."

Well, I would respond to them: "Tell this to my many thousands of patients who have had their cancers get controlled, in some cases going into long-term remission—thanks largely to changes in diet, coupled with non-traditional treatment methods."

Just as forcefully, I would stand tall, in telling such lame prognosticators: "Tell this to the many cancer patients who received no benefit whatsoever from standard, poisonous treatments—or to the surviving relatives of cancer patients who needlessly died without being given the opportunity to at least try potentially effective anti-cancer, high-alkaline diets."

Many practitioners of alternative medicine genuinely hope that widely acclaimed organizations that strive to vilify us aren't doing so primarily out of motivation for the almighty dollar. Yet, sadly, based on what I've seen, many of us concede that essentially "Big Brother is out to get us, because our sensible systems threaten their livelihoods."

Effectiveness Remains in Question

Amid these steadily intensifying controversies, numerous news articles and scientific reports indicate that while there may be some increase in the body's alkalinity from the alkaline diet, any potential benefits are minimal at best. Meantime, some prognosticators even proclaim that cancer does not necessarily thrive in acidic environments, but rather it's the disease and its tumors that actually create buildups of acids in those areas of the body. As if striving to push this proverbial dagger further into the heart of the alternative medicine industry, the American Institute for Cancer Research in 2012 proclaimed that within the body it's "virtually impossible" to create a less acidic environment. Heaping on even more criticism as if in a concerted and organized effort to disclaim homeopathy, others allied to Big Pharma and Big Food have labeled such diets as "extreme."

To such claims, I would say: "I'm pleased to report to the American public and to consumers worldwide that by taking effective measures and treatments to control and to minimize acidity within the body—coupled with the elimination of sugars in the diet, combined with varieties of other treatments, I have successfully eliminated or controlled the cancers of many hundreds of patients. Some cases result in the cessation of cancer growth, or enough positive progress to put tumors into dormancy."

All along, of course, much more scientific research needs to be done. Also, the survival rate of my patients is not 100 percent—although far higher than the standard 5-year mark of 2.1 percent of stage IV cancer patients treated with standard protocol therapy. With just as much forcefulness, I also stress that an alkaline diet should never be considered as or touted as a "cure." While embracing a "whole-body" approach to potentially effective medicine, my clinic would never recommend a blanket, similar, universal alkaline diet for all patients.

Fully mindful of these factors, all homeopaths collectively need to acknowledge that some Websites and publications might be committing "diet fraud." Although not always necessarily criminal in nature, numerous Web pages reportedly require subscription fees before giving consumers regularly issued information on alkaline diets. Such services are among factors that motivate seasoned health professionals to warn consumers that they should avoid diets that severely restrict or even prohibit eating certain fats or carbohydrates.

Adding further to the confusion, some Websites or publications even insist that they'll reveal the anti-cancer, alkaline diet "secrets" being purposely withheld from the public by the scientific community.

Mindful of such concerns, those of us who profess the benefits of limiting acidic food also need to take great care to avoid generating vitamin and mineral deficiencies—conditions that could result in health complications. Eating far too much of certain foods on a non-stop, regular basis could generate an unbalanced diet, potentially causing severe decreases in essential fatty acids.

Food Types

A wide variety of published reports and scientific research list various foods as either primarily forming acids or increasing alkalinity within the body. Amazingly, there seems to be no universal and reliable single source, recognized by homeopaths and dietitians as listing specific food groups within these categories. However, here is a primary listing of overall food groups often found in each:

Acid-Forming foods: Pastas, crackers, fish, margarine, lentils, ice cream, several popular artificial sweeteners, soda pop, poultry, candy, peanut butter, pastries, alcohol, pastry, pasteurized milk, most nuts and seeds, eggs, commercially produced cheese, poultry, noodles, coffee, most processed grains, lentils, most prescription drugs, and most legumes. Listing many of these foods as acid-forming might confuse many people who are eager to maintain anti-cancer diets. For instance some foods often listed as healthful or with antioxidant attributes are often considered as acid-forming, such as fish, most nuts, seeds, most legumes and lentils. Faced with such oxymorons, some consumers might find themselves exclaiming: "It seems that many foods are considered healthful, while also being blamed as potentially cancer-causing. It's all so confusing!" Understandably, who could blame people for feeling that way? Perhaps the best strategy would be to take a sensible approach, working closely with a homeopath or dietitian skilled at helping to address your specific needs.

Alkaline-Forming Foods: These include soy sauce, olive oil, raw milk, most raw vegetables, sauerkraut, green tea, most raw fruits, wheatgrass, sea vegetables, sprouts, apple cider vinegar, herbs, honey, herbal tea, stevia, and molasses.

Scientists believe that many types of food derived from animals tend to form acids within the body—everything from eggs to poultry, meat and fish. The human body's digestive process generates acidic byproducts from these foods. Numerous homeopaths contend that buildups of these byproducts tend to lessen any potential alkalinity that these same foods might generate.

Elements Good for pH Balance

Many vitamins and minerals are deemed by homeopaths as excellent tools in helping to bring the body's pH levels into balance—and thereby decreasing the probability of cancer. One

of these attributes mentioned most often is Vitamin D, critical
in assisting the body's efforts to absorb essential levels of bone-
building, cancer-fighting calcium. But adequate food sources
for vitamin D are extremely rare. Fish is among food sources
mentioned most frequently as having high Vitamin D content.

Another source deemed as adequate and healthful levels of
exposure is the sun. But the damage to the earth's ozone layer,
increasing dangerous ultra-violate levels that can cause skin
cancers, has motivated people from many cultures worldwide to
become "sun dodgers."

Still, the potential benefits that Vitamin D can generate in
extending life by assisting in calcium absorption are legendary.
People in high-mountain cultures around the world are believed
to live long lives as overall groups thanks to the high content of
calcium in their primary water—glacially fed springs supplied by
sources enriched by this mineral. These long-lived calcium-rich
cultures include the Tibetans, the Hunzas of Pakistan, Georgians in
Russia, Armenians, the Bamas of China, and the Titicacas Indians
of Peru.

At sea level, the Okinawa region of Japan is expected to have
by far the world's highest per-capita population of people older
than 100. High levels of coral calcium within the Okinawa drinking
water system have been credited with enriching the health of
people who live there, the incidences of cancer extremely low.

Emboldened and encouraged by such long-lived, naturally
occurring dietary lifestyles, homeopaths have helped develop
dietary supplements deemed high in Vitamin D, calcium and
magnesium. Some publications strongly recommend consumers
look for supplements listing calcium as "high-grade" or "marine
harvested." These products usually are sold with high Vitamin D
content, necessary in fortifying or bolstering the body's effective

absorption of calcium. When using marine-harvested varieties, people who are highly allergic to shellfish or large shrimp should use caution. People with such allergies should ingest such products only under the supervision of a medical professional.

Saliva Testing

Some homeopaths use saliva tests to determine if the body's apparent alkaline range falls within what many health professionals consider the optimal range of 7.0 to 7.5 on the pH scale. However, patients who get such results are cautioned to avoid assuming that their cancers will naturally die as a result of such alkaline levels.

Always remember that the bodily area immediately around a tumor sometimes remains acidic even though the rest of the person has healthful alkaline levels. Thus, while some natural treatment practitioners believe a healthy pH-balanced diet can greatly assist in an overall comprehensive cancer treatment regimen, other solutions will become necessary.

To address this condition, doctors sometimes use a specialized, highly technical non-dietary Cesium High pH Therapy process for alkalizing the biological environment immediately around cancer cells. These treatments involve "caesium," sometimes called "cesium," a silvery-gold alkali metal chemical element often deemed valuable in Ph-balancing cancer treatments.

Chapter 31 Summary

Many people striving to avoid cancer or recover from the disease embrace "alkaline diets" because cancer dies in such environments—while thriving in acidity. Yet many standard oncologists and numerous major organizations insist there is no conclusive scientific evidence that such meal plans prevent or eliminate cancer. These same prognosticators also insist that tumors actually create the acidic environments within the bodily regions where the cancer thrives. However, based on nearly a half century of professional experience, as a doctor I strongly believe that such dietary protocols make a substantial difference in enabling the recoveries of many cancer patients. Foods sometimes deemed as acid-forming and thus to be avoided or eaten in minimal quantities include artificial sweeteners, crackers, margarine, soda pop, poultry, candy, peanut butter, pastries and numerous other crops. By contrast, foods considered as alkaline-forming and thus recommended during alkaline diets include soy sauce, olive oil, raw milk, most raw vegetables and numerous other foods herbs, honey, herbal tea and molasses. Homeopaths consider various elements including Vitamin D and calcium as excellent in helping the body maintain an ideal pH balance.

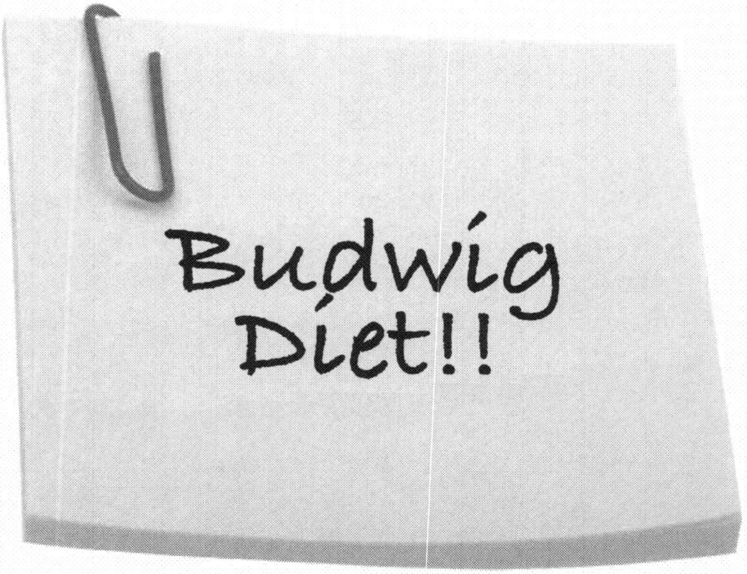
Budwig
Diet!!

Chapter 32

The Budwig
Diet Controversy

Any comprehensive discussion of anti-cancer meal programs requires at least some mention of the highly controversial "Budwig Diet"—plus several other meal programs.

Countless people worldwide, perhaps tens of thousands of them, swear to the effectiveness of the relatively simple Budwig meal program in successfully managing, controlling or possibly eliminating their cancers.

Despite its widespread popularity, many people have not heard of this controversial diet developed by German author and biochemist Johanna Budwig in the early 1950s. Although there are various other criteria involved, the Budwig Diet consists primarily of basic foods eaten together several times daily:

Flaxseed Oil: Colorless and odorless, this edible food is derived from flax plants. Some scientists believe that the effective attributes of this oil have a relatively short shelf life, even when stored in cool environments.

Cottage cheese: These are mixed with the oil. (Some sources also list milk as an ingredient in addition to cottage cheese. You should check the Budwig Diet's official, authorized Websites to find accurate information on this aspect.)

Fruits: These can be added to the oil-cottage cheese mixture to add flavor. Participants eat meals high in fruits, vegetables and fiber.

Simultaneously while eating these recommended food mixtures and combinations several times daily, participants must avoid meats, sugar, salad oil, margarine and butter.

At least according to reports issued by the American Cancer Society, Budwig claimed that following at least three months on her diet some patients felt much better, and their tumors had either shrunk or disappeared. Encouraged by these apparent results, high demand from people interested in the Budwig Diet seems to be continuing. Many people first learn of this food regimen from friends, relatives or acquaintances. Internet search engines are filled with numerous independent, unaffiliated Websites where many people swear to the diet's effectiveness. Numerous sites feature self-written stories of people who claim they had suffered from stage IV cancers before their symptoms disappeared due to dedicated Budwig Diet regimens.

Specific cases chronicling people who say they were cured involve: metastasized prostate cancer and cancers of the pancreas, breast, brain, and other cancers.

The American Cancer Society has proclaimed that any "cure" or positive results from the Budwig Diet have never been proven. At least according to some publications, scientists in limited studies have generated inclusive results when experimenting on rats. And although limited research has indicated the Budwig Diet might reduce the risk of prostate cancer, additional study is necessary to generate conclusive results.

Budwig Diet History

Budwig concluded that lots of us damage our health by eating far too many oils that have been chemically altered. Her research found that many people fail to consume adequate and essential levels of omega-3 and omega-6 fatty acids. She blamed modern food manufacturers for causing this problem, loading preservatives into natural oils that otherwise would easily spoil. To correct this problem Budwig insisted that consumers everywhere should eat more natural healthy oils.

In Budwig's view, the body cannot produce prostaglandins without the essential omega-3 and omega-6 fatty acids. This would be a potentially critical deficiency because prostaglandins serve a vital role in handling the chemically-generated biological communication among cells. Budwig developed the diet in an attempt to counteract or reverse these deficiencies, fortifying cell membranes and also enabling the body to more efficiently pump life-giving oxygen into cells.

When trying to find the ideal foods for her diet, Budwig identified cottage cheese primarily due to its ability to enable the body to easily and readily absorb the essential but missing fatty acids—particularly in combination with the food's sulfur-based proteins. To handle that aspect Budwig chose flaxseed, which she deemed the most potent source of necessary fatty acids. Ultimately, by combining cottage cheese with flaxseed oil, the result was a water-soluble food that the body easily absorbs.

Adding additional firepower in battling cancer, from Budwig's view, combining these foods also greatly assisted the body's ability to use essential elements in fighting cancer by making prostaglandins—particularly the minerals zinc and magnesium, plus vitamins C and B3 and B6.

At least according to Budwig's scientific papers and various articles chronicling her work, trying to eat flaxseed oil alone in an effort to prevent or control cancer was not nearly as effective as ingesting it with the high-sulfur proteins found in cottage cheese.

Budwig reported that while initially researching the fatty acids issue, before selecting foods for her anti-cancer diet, she had continually found a mysterious greenish-yellow substance inside blood of people with cancer or individuals who were becoming ill. Among many of these same people, and subsequent patients, Budwig reported that the strange materials had disappeared within the bodies of patients who had faithfully used her diet for at least three consecutive months.

Budwig Fought for Patient's Rights

Budwig's claim of positive results naturally incurred the wrath of big businesses that had steered away from natural foods. Manufacturers of major foods slammed her efforts, particularly margarine producers. Without saying so in such specific words, these corporations were essentially portraying her as a buffoon for even daring to question and to admonish their steadily increasing practice of altering oils for preservation, and to speed up food deliveries.

For this very reason, even though her diet might remain suspect in the eyes of many Big Pharma and Big Food officials today, Budwig should be considered a hero. Finally during the mid-1900s concerned consumers started standing up against reckless and selfish major manufacturers and distributors. Although lacking household-name recognition these days, she played a significant role in enabling the public to realize there "is a better way—or at least there can be a better way—when it comes to eating healthy foods."

James W. Forsythe, M.D., H.M.D.

Even today, many consumers fail to realize that at least one prominent doctor eventually started denying Budwig access to a research facility that she previously used. Rather than keeping quiet, leading the way for the increased popularity of her own healthy food regimen and perhaps for other anti-cancer food remedies to follow, Budwig began announcing results of her scientific research. To do this, she wrote about the issue and spent more time working with patients within clinical settings.

Is This Worth the Risk?

As a homeopath and even when practicing solely as an oncologist, I have no direct experience recommending the Budwig Diet or monitoring any apparent results of cancer patients who have chosen to try this food regimen on their own initiative.

Needless to say, this is a touchy subject. From my view as a homeopath, patients have a right to choose their own treatment regimens, particularly natural remedies shunned by mainstream oncologists. Yet there are obvious risks when depending solely on such a rigid, one-size-fits-all diet, especially without the direct care and supervision of a certified medical professional.

Keenly aware of these issues, I give specific advice to any patient who might consider the Budwig Diet: "Do so at your own risk, and realize you might fail to get any positive results. Then, while undergoing the diet, some medical experts might argue that you're failing to get certain vital nutrients that might help speed up your recovery. Worsening matters, without getting direct professional attention to your cancer, you might put your health in extremely serious jeopardy."

Despite such potential drawbacks, at least the Budwig Diet gives some patients potential hope—particularly when discovering the many supposed success stories littered across the Internet.

Throughout my medical career, I have never had any of my many thousands of patients tell me: "Doctor, I'm trying the Budwig Diet. What do you think?"

When and if that ever happens, I would never tell the person flat-out to stop the Budwig Diet regimen. I also would avoid any attempt to belittle the person, never even entertaining the idea of labeling people who try such treatments as "flaky" or "foolish." Disturbingly, though, I have little doubt that patients who casually mention to their doctors that "I'm trying the Budwig Diet," would get negative responses, particularly from practitioners of standard allopathic medicine, and especially from oncologists.

As a cancer patient, when and if you tell your doctor that you're trying the Budwig Diet, remain forthright enough to inform this person of your decision if that's your choice. If and when your doctor tries to belittle you, argues that you should stop using the Budwig Diet or insists that you should never attempt such regimens, always remember that ultimately you have the right to make your own health care decisions.

So, there is no reason to get into a heated argument when and if this issue ever arises with your doctor. Remain calm, and refuse to allow any conflict to intensify. Remember, cancer patients need to avoid unnecessary stress.

Carefully Study the Budwig Issue

Before deciding whether to undergo a Budwig Diet regimen, be sure to conduct as much in-depth research as you can on the issue, fully mindful of the fact that some Websites are flat-out bogus—filled with false information. If numerous people on a single diet make what seem like sensationally positive claims about their Budwig Diet results, you should proceed with caution.

With just as much urgency, you should attempt to find

and chronicle people who failed to get any positive results. Budwig died in 2002 at age 94, but numerous publications or Websites give more in-depth information on the many specifics of implementing the diet. These publications or sites list specific amounts of cottage cheese and flaxseed oil, how to blend them in certain types of machines, and the many things "to do" and to "avoid." Some Websites including BudwigCenter.com offer free downloads of the "Budwig Diet Guide."

Chapter 32 Summary

The controversial anti-cancer Budwig Diet protocol that mandates eating cottage cheese mixed with flaxseed oil while avoiding certain foods has many people swear to its effectiveness—but some doctors and medical organizations insist there is no scientific proof that this cures or controls cancer. The late German author and biochemist Johanna Budwig developed the diet, believing that many cancers come from unhealthful, people-made oils. She believed that the cottage cheese and flaxseed oil mixture provided the best way to easily and effectively get essential anti-cancer elements into the body. Today's oncologists likely would scoff at any declaration by cancer patients declaring that they're on a Budwig Diet, urging these people to avoid such "quackery." All along, my clinic has no experience on this diet's apparent effects, so I'm unable to recommend this diet. Nonetheless, all patients should have a right to choose and dictate their own treatment preferences.

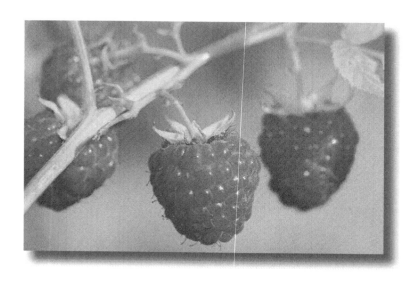

Chapter 33

Other Issues

Besides the Budwig Diet and the various other antioxidants discussed earlier, a wide variety of specific foods, meal strategies and even "negative foods" need to be listed to help cancer patients get a comprehensive idea of the many "positives and negatives" they face. Among them:

Ellagic acid: This naturally occurring anti-cancer compound occurs in many foods, particularly cranberries, pomegranates, blueberries, pecans, blackberries, walnuts, and strawberries. Overall, these are foods containing a high-density reddish color. Mindful of these attributes, some dietitians insist that their clients "go for the reds and deep purples" when eating fruit—particularly high-density red raspberries, which reportedly boast at least six times more of this fantastic natural substance than any other food. Dietitians claim at least 46 fruits and nuts contain ellagic acid. Technically, on a molecular level, these foods include nuts and fruit that contain the healthful ellagitannins, which the human body converts to ellagic acid. Homeopaths deem these attributes so powerful that some supplement producers strive to include this substance in their products. As far back as the 1970s scientists started researching the potential benefits of ellagitannins. At least one study at the Medical University of South Carolina's Hollings Cancer Institute indicated that people can significantly prevent their chances of developing cancer just by eating at least one cup of red raspberries daily—or the equivalent of 40 milligrams of ellagitannins. Results became just as impressive among people already suffering from cancer. At least according to these findings, ellagic acid proves effective in slowing the growth of cancers of the esophagus, pancreas, prostate, colon, cervix and breast. Even greater reason for optimism came when higher-than-normal levels of this incredible substance killed cancer cells. Subsequent studies elsewhere generated similar results, also generating conclusions that ellagic acid fights aggressively against leukemia and melanoma. Ideally, researchers studying cancer want to find substances—particularly natural remedies—that cause "G-arrest," wrecking the ability of cancer cells to divide and thus grow. Researchers also found that besides destroying cancer ellagic acid: serves as an antioxidant, sweeping away free radicals; helps kick immunity into healthy and effective levels; fights viruses; prevents DNA and toxic carcinogens from binding; and cleans away toxins from enzymes within the liver. Similar to Web pages touting the Budwig Diet, numerous sites chronicle the positive claims of cancer patients who insist their disease was wiped out or seriously hampered thanks to foods rich with ellagitannins. Even so, consumers also are cautioned to be wary of unscrupulous merchants who sell red raspberry extracts that have lost their potency—sometimes amid lengthy storage periods in warehouses. Thus, buyers eager to get the most benefit possible from ellagic acid should deal only with reputable manufacturers and distributors that are highly recommended by real, live consumers—preferably people whose cancers went into remission or disappeared. Many consumers like the fact that ellagic acid is inexpensive compared to high-priced Big Pharma medications that usually pose extremely serious potential side effects.

The CAAT Protocol: First developed in 1944, an acronym for "Controlled Amino Acid Therapy," this powerful nutrition and diet approach is sometimes used with good results—particularly among patients with advanced cancers. Some homeopaths oversee this protocol on patients who have undergone radiation and/ or conventional chemo. Numerous patients also undergo CAAT Protocols without ever undergoing the typical standard poisonous or highly dangerous standard-medicine treatments. This unique strategy involves the use of three primary factors: specific "phytochemicals," a term for natural chemical compounds; a strict diet regimen; and certain pre-designated amino acids. For a CAAT Protocol to work effectively, the patient also must avoid certain foods or supplements that health professionals deem likely to form or feed cancer. Essentially, the doctors use this complex strategy to starve cancers to death, while also preventing its formation. The protocol first developed by the late Angelo P. John, a cancer researcher and molecular biologist, usually lasts from six months to nine months. According to various sources and published reports, the CAAT protocol attacks cancer in four ways: wrecks the body's ability to produce specific amino acids that cancers need to replicate; lessens the body's ability to generate and use hormones that would otherwise help cancers grow; prevents the growth of new blood vessels, such as occur occasionally in areas of inflammation, thereby blocking the ability of cancers to form in those locations; and hampers the "glycolysis" process within cancer cells, a metabolic system that converts glucose into pyruvic acid, critical in supplying energy to living cells through what scientists call the "citric acid cycle." Also called "Kerbs cycle," this process, unless inhibited, creates the lactic acid that the muscles and cancers need when oxygen isn't present. While very low in protein and carbohydrate, the protocol's diet strictly limits the types and amounts of fats. Some consumers try to get these attributes in supplement form. But only the A.P. John Cancer Institute in Connecticut can distribute its propriety blend of amino acids and give certified guidance. Consumers or their physicians can contact the institute at (877) 260-1588, or via its Website, APJohnCancerInstitute.org.

Exotic Botanicals: Primarily from South American rainforests, food products within this segment include medicinal teas and herbs touted as having anti-cancer attributes. One of the best known is derived from the Lapacho tree that grows in Paraguay, Argentina and Brazil. The bark of Lapachos is often used to make teas deemed highly effective in fighting or preventing cancer. Lapachos, also called Taheebo or Pau D'Arco or even the "Divine Tree," is used for Tajy tea. The Lapacho is derived from the Tabeabubia genre that has at least 100 species, only a handful used for medicinal purposes. Hailed for its many attributes from antioxidant to anti-inflammatory and analgesic, Lapacho Tea is credited by some researchers for stimulating red blood cell production. According to various news stories and scientific reports, of the nine patients in a scientific study who were given capsules of "lapachol," the active ingredient from in Lapacho Tea, three of the people went into complete remission from the disease. Controversy seems to erupt at least on a mild scale because Big Pharma has been unable to clinically prove the beneficial effects of the tea's primary components. Thus, major pharmaceutical companies were unable to isolate effective concentrations of Lapachos' active ingredient, to the point that such processing could be patented in order to generate corporate profit. South American physicians insist that they get better results when administering Lapacho treatments as a tea rather than when using the isolated active ingredients. Brazilian physicians started getting what they described as phenomenal results—with some patients going into remission in as little as four weeks, according to some news accounts. Positive media reports stirred up such enthusiasm that until scientists could complete comprehensive studies, government officials ordered a news blackout. Some observers still insist that more comprehensive research is necessary, particularly regarding specifically how Lapacho Tea apparently destroys or damages cancer on a biological level. According to some published reports, this tea uncouples specific mitochondrial functions within cancer cells—wrecking their oxygen-processing capacity, while leaving non-cancerous cells unharmed. Understandably, some consumer advocates and medical professionals urge cancer patients to seek out Lapacho Tea only from legitimate sources. The potential for wide-scale, debilitating fraud exists due to the huge demand for this product. Journalists have chronicled instances where the bark of Lapacho trees was not properly harvested or prepared. Some companies including Vibrant Life Vitamins claim to generate Lapacho that's medicinally active and high-quality in capsule form. High doses are recommended for cancer patients, at least two capsules hourly throughout the day starting with a minimum five of these pills in the morning. Some producers insist that consumers will either experience no results, or they'll start feeling better within three weeks. While these doses are considered high for any herb or medication, even higher doses of Lapacho are recommended by some health care professionals amid instances where tumors are decreasing in size; the strategy here is to take increased amounts of this substance until the cancer disappears.

LifeOne™ Formula: Hailed by its practitioners as an effective non-toxic cancer treatment, this liquid formula has also been recently touted as effective in treating AIDS/HIV. Scientists developed this product by mixing a variety of effective substances including organic selenium, medicinal mushrooms, flavonoids, various powerful herbs, phytochemicals, resveratrol, lecithin, and phosphatidycholine, a class of phospholipids—the major components of cell membranes. Among the many reported powerful attributes of LifeOne™ Formula: kills viruses; improves cell functions; and balances hormones, putting the immunity system back in balance. Thanks to these attributes, LifeOne™ has been credited by a number of publications with destroying various types of cancer cells, including those of the ovaries, colon, breast, cervix and prostate, plus acute Promyelocytic leukemia. Although LifeOne™ is taken orally as a liquid, and therefore can be considered part of the "diet," it's not administered in large doses such as by the cup. Instead, under standard protocol, it's taken during the first month three times daily in two-tablespoon doses. Thus, when under this phase of the standard regimen the person ingests nearly a half cup of the liquid daily. The initial month is followed by an 11-month routine where the patient takes one tablespoon, three times daily. Dr. James A. Howenstine, a LifeOne Therapy expert, has been quoted as saying that patients who eliminate high-glycemic foods like wheat, white potatoes, pasta, corn and bananas from their diets, and also restrict their sugar intake have experienced a quicker and more effective response. In addition, people who have not had radiation or chemo often get the best results. To see patient testimonials on this product, visit LifeOne.org.

N-Tense: Besides the beneficial cat's claw mentioned earlier, this herbal formulation features "graviola"—also known as "soursop," the beneficial fruit of a flowering evergreen tree that grows in South America, Central America, Mexico and Cuba. While half of N-Tense is comprised of graviola the other ingredients besides cat's claw—other powerful South American rainforest botanicals—are bitter melon, guacatonga, mullaca, espinheira santa, mutamba and vassourinha. A 2011 "Nutrition and Cancer" article said that laboratory tests reveal evidence indicating that extracts from the graviola fruit inhibit human breast cancer growth within mice, but more tests need to be done on people. For now, scientists have chronicled at least 20 research tests where graviola killed cancer cells in laboratory studies. The only company that produces N-Tense, Rain-Tree Nutrition Inc, makes no claims regarding its impact on cancer. However, numerous people who have used this herb formulation insist that it has significantly helped control or eliminate their cancers.

Ham: Anyone concerned about maintaining good health, and especially cancer, should avoid eating ham—particularly cured or processed. Consistent studies indicate that the consumption of red meats is a precursor for cancer. Many hams sold in the United States, particularly those shipped and offered in cans, are processed—usually meaning that chemicals or excessive salts have been added. Although there seems to be no conclusive evidence that ham causes cancer, numerous homeopaths strongly suggest that you avoid such selections. Lots of people seem to enjoy ham mostly during holidays like Thanksgiving, Christmas and Easter when this meat is often serves as a mainstay at public buffets or family parties. Many health professionals might argue that just one serving of ham certainly will never cause any long-term harm. However, although studies seem incomplete on this issue, perhaps consuming ham coupled with other negative lifestyle decisions could combine to generate cancers. This becomes apparent when considering the fact that within the United States lots of dry hams are loaded with sugars added during processing. Additional potential health problems emerge when processors cram salt into the hams as a flavor enhancer. Topping this off, according to a 2006 article in the "World Journal of Gastroenterology," the nitrates in hams causes this food's amino acids to degrade. Certain conditions can cause this transition to form nitrosamines, chemical compounds that most scientists universally agree are carcinogenic. Without listing scientific sources, numerous publications claim that various production processes form nitrosamine in a variety of foods, including certain beers, fish and cheeses. Such reports would be reckless unless backed by sound, verifiable research. Yet consumers have a right to be concerned. All along, hams—particularly canned varieties—undoubtedly fall high on any homeopath's list of potential offenders.

Hot dogs: Within the mainstream public mindset within the United States, hot dogs are generally considered "All-America," right up there with mom, apple pie and hamburgers. Sure enough, to the average consumer this might seem like an innocent, innocuous food that everyone should appreciate. After all, these foods are standard fare at baseball games, often hailed as "America's favorite pastime." Yet don't be fooled, at least from a health standpoint. A huge percentage of hot dogs sold at public events and in grocery stores are highly processed meats—often affectionately called everything from "frankfurters" to "sausages" and "weenies." Usually made of beef, pork or chicken, hot dogs go way back in the American culture as a favorite "finger food," usually wrapped in warm buns and slathered with sauces, relishes, hot dogs and mustard. Due partly to the relatively easy and fast preparation process, hot dogs motivate entrepreneurs to operate food stands on corners of busy streets in many major metropolitan areas.

James W. Forsythe, M.D., H.M.D.

Without question these foods are engrained in the American culture, widely considered as highly safe and even nutritious. Yet many homeopaths urge their patients to steer clear of such temptations because the vast majority of hot dogs are highly processed. Some health professionals worry that hot dogs may contain dangerously high levels of salt, potentially causing hypertension and even stroke. The apparent possible dangers increase even more, particularly among many food venues that singe or burn hot dog skins on grills—a potential precursor, as discussed earlier, in causing highly dangerous cancer-causing free radicals. Usually without any indication on packaging, many hot dogs are preserved with sodium nitrate. Although this can sometimes prevent certain bacteria from growing, and thus serve as a preservative, sodium nitrate is sometimes considered highly toxic to humans. When consumed in excessive amounts, elements of high sodium nitrate toxicity can cause the liver to work far too hard, clearing a potential pathway for the formation of cancer within the body. Food processors might argue that nitrates are a normal and harmless part of the natural food chain, so widespread it's found in most vegetables. Yet high concentrations of sodium nitrate excessively processed into meats like hot dogs should spark concern among consumers. Some doctors concede that high concentrations of sodium nitrates are fatal. An "International Journal of Epidemiology" article in the year 2000 indicated that sodium nitrates have a possibility of becoming carcinogenic due to this substance's interaction with the acidic environment of the human stomach—similar to when free radicals get formed when over-cooking meats on grills. Another dangerous and potentially carcinogenic process mentioned in this article and other publications has been the chemical transformation of sodium nitrate during the meat curing process. This often involves what chefs and food manufacturers call "smoking," for the primary purpose of preserving, flavoring, or cooking meats. Although the smoking of foods is a common and widely accepted procedure, various medical and government publications strongly suggest that overall this curing procedure contains or generates carcinogens. On a scientific level, some experts say, smoking meats creates what biologists call "polycyclic aromatic hydrocarbon," highly suspected as a dangerous hidden cancer-causing atomic structure. As a result, many homeopaths warn that foods containing these substances—particularly hot dogs—sharply increase the risk of gastrointestinal cancer, malignant and often eventually fatal conditions of the anus, stomach, esophagus, bowels, pancreas and the bile system. Even amid such concerns, some health or medical organizations including the National Cancer Institute emphasize that studies of wide populations have not generated conclusive evidence of a verifiable link between cancer in people and smoked meats. A wide variety of foods are smoked, particularly those high in proteins including cheeses, various fish species including salmon, jerky, and fruits such as prunes. Although the vast majority of medical professionals refrain from flat-out saying "do not eat these foods," some consumers might choose to avoid them while carefully studying the risks. A 1998 FDA publication indicated that people with histories of suffering migraine headaches sometimes experience these excruciatingly painful episodes after eating foods such as hot dogs that contain sodium nitrate. Even for consumers who have never suffered migraines, avoiding hot dogs might be a effective step in minimizing the possibility of cancer.

Bacon: This popular food is generated by curing meats from pigs. To issue a blanket, uniform statement that "bacon causes cancer" likely would incur the wrath of this entire industry.

Nonetheless, largely because bacon is cured and processed, it should be of concern to anyone diligent about preventing or controlling cancer. For this reason, people who choose to avoid bacon should remain fully cognizant that it's often used as a spice or flavor enhancer in a wide variety of recipes including salads—sometimes added in a form called "bacon bits." Food manufacturers also occasionally use ground bacon as an additive in a variety of products, including certain dressings. So, people who want to avoid bacon should carefully inspect food packaging labels. All along, to imply that "bacon causes cancer" might be considered reckless, particularly if such a statement comes from a medical professional. Like hot dogs and ham, there is no conclusive overall scientific evidence that bacon causes cancer—although it usually contains the attributes that many homeopaths believe increases the likelihood of getting the disease. Even so, a 2007 Columbia University study suggested that obstructive pulmonary disease is sometimes the result of eating cured meats like bacon. Compounding matters outside the realm of cancer, the risk of getting both diabetes and heart disease increase when eating meats such as bacon that are cured by adding chemical preservatives, salting or smoking, according to a 2010 Harvard School of Public Health study. Bacon usually fries in its own grease, which has very little nutritional value and high fat content. Multiplying these concerns, some dietary listings indicate that four pieces of cooked bacon have the equivalent of 1.92 grams of salt. That's nearly a third of the suggested maximum daily sodium intake recommended in some regions, including the United Kingdom—which tells people not to exceed six grams daily. Excessive salt consumption if often blamed for causing everything from hypertension to stroke, enlargement of the heart, high blood pressure, stomach cancers, and edema, an excessive and potentially dangerous buildup of body fluid.

Katsup: Although this product, sometimes spelled "catsup" has been a mainstay or primary staple within the typical diets of many Americans, many brands are sweetened with either high-fructose corn syrup, considered by many health professionals as a potential precursor for cancer. This food also is sometimes sweetened by sugar, universally shunned by many consumers who want to prevent or manage the disease. Besides their notorious associations with cancer, high-fructose corn syrup and white sugar also are collectively and individually often blamed as major contributors to obesity. Following the publication of some health publications and especially "Wheat Belly," some producers of famous brand-name catsups stopped using sugar or high-fructose corn syrup. Some plastic, bottle-shaped packages started boasting "no corn syrup." Did this recent change result from an increased public concern sparked by health publications that cited the notoriety of these ingredients? Had overall catsup sales temporarily decreased, before manufacturers made this change? Still, many brands still are sweetened by one or both of the potentially dangerous substances. So, consumers determined to avoid sugar or high-fructose corn syrup should check labels, or ask restaurant servers if catsup that's delivered in a cup "on the side" contains these substances. Additionally, some food service venues including snack stands at movie theaters occasionally have metal pumps available for buyers to put their own catsup on—you guessed it—hot dogs. These catsup dispensers contain no nutritional-content labels. So, you probably would need to ask the cinema's personnel if the catsup contains high-fructose corn syrup or white sugar; but those employees likely would not have an answer. Some publications claim that catsup contains the antioxidant lycopene, a bright red pigment of the carotenoid and carotene crop sectors—previously shown to have anti-cancer attributes.

Millet: Since we have millet as among primary options as substitutes for wheat, a basic description is in order. People with gluten intolerance often become encouraged when learning it lacks this substance. Just as impressive from an anti-cancer perspective, millet also contains zinc, magnesium, potassium, calcium and iron. Numerous millet varieties exist, all from small-seeded grasses grown mostly in semi-arid tropics, particularly in Asia and Africa—especially in Niger, India and Nigeria. Besides proso millet, usually grown for use as bird seed, the other primary species of this crop are: finger millet, grown primarily in Asia and Africa, upper elevations of the Himalayans and particularly the Ethiopian Highlands, it's often used as a cereal that has vital amino acids or proteins; and foxtail millet, sometimes called "Italian millet," "German millet," or "Chinese millet," it's most important in East Asia.

Chapter 33 Summary

Numerous food- or herb-related anti-cancer treatments receive little mention in the mainstream media. But they're worth mentioning due to their possible or apparent effectiveness. These include: Ellagic acid treatments, administered via a compound believed by some scientists as a cancer destroyer that fights viruses, helps immunity, clears free radicals; and various other cancer-fighting chores; the Controlled Amino Acid Therapy or CAAT protocol, thought to destroy the ability of cancer cells to replicate; LifeOne™ Formula, a mixture of anti-cancer substances taken in tablespoon doses for at least one year; N-Tense, mixtures of cat's claw and other anti-cancer "graviola" fruits from flowering plants in Cuba, Mexico, Central America and South America. All along, some homeopaths urge patients to avoid processed meats sometimes deemed carcinogenic including ham, hot dogs, bacon and katsup.

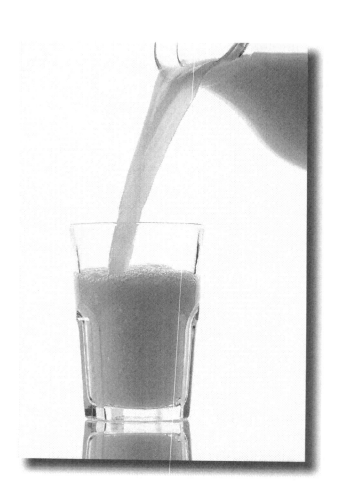

Chapter 34

Juicing

A highly controversial yet potentially effective method of efficiently ingesting massive quantities of antioxidants and anti-cancer foods involves juicing.

Made popular partly thanks to the diligence of the late good-health advocate Jack LaLanne, juicing involves the use of machines to extract juices from vegetables, fruits and sometimes nutrient supplements.

Many people embracing this lifestyle also use plenty of whey protein powder in their juices to ensure the body gets adequate amino acids necessary for energy. The process generates pros and cons, adding to the disagreements between those who insist juicing has no definitive health benefits whatsoever and people who swear to its effectiveness. Among their stances:

Pros: These people insist the body gets massive does of critical vitamins, including anti-cancer citric acids, antioxidants from specific vegetables, and ample energy-boosting proteins to help strengthen the immunity system. Although meat generally is shunned by many good-health advocates, some "juicers"—people who enjoy this lifestyle—choose to include bits of turkey, chicken and non-red meats, and even some fish. When taken several times daily, these health advocates say, the proteins, high vitamin content and essential minerals keep hunger pangs in check—ultimately resulting in weight loss. Meantime, boosted by these steady doses of proteins, these people say they're better able to exercise and to build muscle. This might prove essential in an overall good-health and anti-cancer regimen, because muscle generally needs the body to expend more calories to maintain its structures. Fats require less calories than muscles, and thus when people build or bulk-up their muscles the overall percentage of fat within in the body often decreases. This in turn, some people say, can result in a decrease in nagging belly fat, the known contributor to various cancers. Many people who use juicers one or more times daily insist they enjoy far more physical energy and suffer cancer in far less frequency than the general population.

Cons: These people cite the fact that no definable, universally acknowledged scientific evidence exists to back the assertion that juicing provides any anti-cancer attributes at all. Along a similar tract, another argument suggests that there's no specific reason to believe that juicing increases or assists markedly in the body's digestion and absorption of critical anti-cancer vitamins, antioxidants and minerals. Worsening matters, there's also a concern that perhaps juicing might actually create the opposite effect from what its proponents strive to achieve—an effective tool in reaching a good, balanced and solid overall personal diet regimen. The fear here hinges on a concern that some people who "juice" will become malnourished, particularly if they start avoiding solid foods altogether. Another key worry stems from the fact that a percentage of people experience "digestive situations" when juicing, particularly as they start such regimens—at least until the body gets accustomed to the soft, drenched, milkshake-like meals. Diarrhea can become a common complaint, particularly in the beginning. Flatulence and a buildup of bodily gasses is a common issue, particularly among people juicing for the first time, perhaps due to the massive simultaneous consumption of large amounts of fruits and vegetables. Lots of juicing advocates insist that these symptoms usually disappear, once the person's digestive tract becomes accustomed to these foods. The Mayo Clinic has announced its finding that there is no scientific conclusion that juicing provides any better food than simply eating the same fruits and vegetables.

Amid these various pros and cons, there's also apparent disagreement on whether juicing creates a positive or negative environment within critical bacteria that line the intestines. Advocates claim that juicing favors and assists such organisms; others disagree, contending there's a chance that critical bacteria might get damaged.

All along, homeopaths might find themselves admitting that indeed no overall conclusive evidence seems to exist on any supposed irrefutable, anti-cancer health benefits from juicing. Even so, how could instantly filling the body with massive simultaneous meals of powerful antioxidants at non-toxic levels possibly do any harm? There apparently has been no conclusive laboratory or scientific tests proving that juicing is harmful.

Ultimately, as long as juicing causes no apparent long-term or serious physical harm, why not enjoy this lifestyle and take advantage of its potential benefits?

Juicing Methods

While a vast majority of juicing is done using electric machines, some people prefer to extract juices from foods via hand. Rather than merely electronic blenders, machines specifically designed for this are called "juicers," available at relatively low cost in many department stores. Expenses can increase for buyers choosing bigger, more elaborate, higher priced machine models or brands—mostly variable-speed, motor-driven devices.

Commercial juicing, the process of producing these foods at health food stores in malls or in specialized restaurants, usually involves processing fruits. Vegetables enter the mix on a commercial level at venues like supermarkets. While these offerings attract many consumers, huge numbers of people enjoy creating their own concoctions at home. The thinking here is, "Why should I rely on a cookie-cutter method, when I can create my own favorites using various amounts of the foods that I like most?" Some consumers also prefer making all their own foods at home anyway.

A wide range of videos, advertisements and books on the subject have either created or resulted in a continuous public health "juicing craze." Nonetheless, although many consumers are familiar with the overall term and process of "juicing," lots of people remain unfamiliar with what the overall process entails, unaware of how they should proceed.

Nevertheless, what might seem potentially difficult or challenging can sometimes emerge as quite easy, when a person eventually tries out juicing for the first time. At least judging from what its advocates proclaim, the process is fairly easy and enjoyable.

Essentially similar to asking a person out on a first date, all it takes to incorporate juicing into your lifestyle is that "initial move." Advocates say that simply buying a machine, before getting and juicing your favorite foods—particularly antioxidants—for good health can spark a desire to enjoy this lifestyle for many years.

James W. Forsythe, M.D., H.M.D.

History and Processes

For hundreds and in some cases thousands of years juicing has been done using everything from barrel-shaped presses to inverted cones for mashing and twisting fruit, and hand-operated grinders. Today's electronic juicers use variations of three processes:

Triturating: To extract maximum amounts of juice, these machines use twin gears. Sauce, purees and dips become possible at lower speeds.

Masticating: These grind and knead foods through a chute, striving to retain more fiber, particularly at slower speeds from a single motor.

Centrifugal: Resembling a grated basket, spinning blades push pulp into receptacles while quickly grinding food.

Before buying an electronic juicer, check which types of processors are available, preferably when displayed side-by-side in a single store. This way it's easier to compare which is more likely to give the result you want—such as pulp-free beverages or juices lacking such heavier substances.

Juice Fasting

As part of what some homeopaths call a "detox diet" or a fasting diet, when "juice fasting" a person consumes only fruits or vegetables for pre-set limited times. The goal is usually to remove toxins from the body, to enable digestive bacteria to strengthen, or to simultaneously achieve both those goals. The juice-fasting process enables people to get at least some nutrition, rather than abstaining from food in an effort to achieve the same health-oriented objectives. Some physicians warn that "juice-fasting" can be dangerous, while also emphasizing that scientists have been unable to find evidence that such strategies truly achieve the desired results. Depending on specific recommendations of various advocates of this process, including some publications, periods of juice fasting can last from a few days to several weeks. Many doctors would worry that going without solid, nutrition-based foods for long periods is tantamount to starving the body of critical elements that people need to live and to maintain good health. From this viewpoint, people who knowingly try juice fasting without any verifiable scientific evidence to back up their efforts are essentially taking their lives into their own hands—largely for no good reason whatsoever. Amid such fasting, the juice is usually not of varieties sold in stores, but rather products that can only be made at home. Besides efforts to control, manage or prevent cancer, the many reasons that people undergo juice-fasting regimens include: eliminating addictions to unhealthful habits like smoking, overeating, or drinking too much soda. According to a variety of publications, others try this strategy as a supposed cure for everything from chronic pain and depression to autoimmune deficiencies and many other diseases. Just like with its potential effect on cancer, however, juice fasting has never been proven as effective in treating these many ailments. Even so, either unaware of such warnings or ignoring them, U.S. consumers sometimes go on lengthy trips to engage in juice-fasting sessions with other people at spas and resorts in other countries including Thailand. Compounding the potential dangers, at least in the eyes of standard doctors, some juice fasters also take laxatives or undergo enemas, hoping to expel waste or "bad bacteria" from their intestines and colons while abstaining from food. The process can become more intensive for those who choose to add psyllium to their juices, hoping to boost the body's absorption of water. Even when such steps are made, the low sodium content of most fruits and vegetables could generate extremely serious headaches, weakness and eventually nausea from salt deficiencies within the body. Rather than face such grave health risks, simply drinking inexpensive pure water can work wonders in helping to naturally push toxins from the body, according to many health professionals—who also consider costly detox diets as highly dangerous.

Smoothies

Unlike most standard substances that undergo juicing, smoothies usually have a thickness and texture similar to milk shakes. Like many juiced foods, smoothes often contain healthy fruits, some with everything from crushed ice to honey, syrups, yogurt or ice cream. Like foods that undergo standard juicing, some smoothies can contain highly nutritious minerals, vitamins and anti-oxidants. The amount of nutrition depends, of course, on what specific foods are included. Many smoothies are generally considered healthy, but those attributes falter or become non-existent when a smoothie contains carcinogens like sugar and artificial sweeteners. Also, unlike regular "juicer" foods that remain relatively unknown to the general public, smoothies have gained widespread acceptance throughout American society—particularly since the late 1960s. By the early 21st Century, smoothies had become part of mainstream restaurant menus including at major food chains like McDonald's. Not to be outdone, many community coffee shops and even international conglomerates like Starbucks® began offering smoothies, too. Such blanket, widespread sales should never appease advocates of anti-cancer diets. When that's your specific goal in deciding whether to buy a smoothie, be sure to ask if it contains antioxidants and whether it has carcinogens like sugar and artificial sweeteners.

Health Shake

Like juiced foods and standard smoothies, health shakes are usually processed in machines, but sometimes have extremely high calorie content, according to "The Daily Plate" publication. Due to the high concentrations of foods like peanut butter and bee pollens, health shakes reportedly may contain even more calories than a standard-size breakfast serving of pancakes or cheese omelets. From the viewpoint of anti-cancer advocates, a health shake—like juiced foods and smoothies—is only beneficial when containing high levels of antioxidants, vitamins and essential cancer-fighting minerals like magnesium and calcium. Rather than merely snacks, some health shakes are used to replace entire meals. Also, largely due to the fact that they're also made in electronic food blenders or grinders, health shakes sometimes are considered as a form of smoothie. A specific type of health shake is sometimes called "green smoothie," loaded with anti-cancer foods, primarily leafy vegetables like broccoli, parsley, collard greens, spinach, and Swiss chard. Besides ice or water, many green smoothies also contain fruits, especially apples, bananas, and oranges.

Chapter 34 Summary

Some consumers and cancer patients believe that the juicing or electronic mixing of foods dense in antioxidants effectively prevents or controls the disease. But prognosticators claim there is no scientific evidence to back such claims. Even so, ingesting such natural antioxidant foods simultaneously in high concentrations could only help rather than hurt the person—but only as long as bodily consumption is below non-toxic levels. Numerous alleged health experts recommend "juice fasting;" people undergo continuous multiple days without eating solid food—drinking juiced mixtures of specific foods like carrots. The goal is to eliminate harmful toxins from the body. But such strategies could be extremely harmful or even fatal, especially when attempted without the guidance of a licensed medical professional. Other variations of juicing include: smoothies, primarily the mixing of helpful fruits; and health shakes, which some practitioners claim are bulk and constitute full meals.

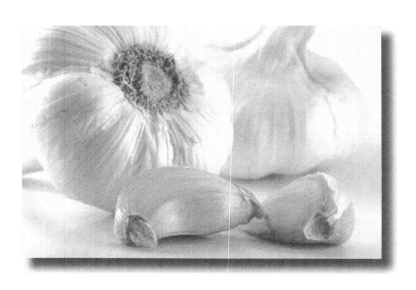

Chapter 35

Garlic Magic

Throughout the ages, many people have claimed that garlic—sometimes hailed as the "Nectar of the Gods"—has miraculous positive health attributes, possibly including strong anti-cancer action. Yet even today such claims remain inconclusive and unproven regarding its impact on the disease.

Even so, according to various reports including a study described in the Proceedings of the National Academy of Sciences claim that garlic increases the body's hydrogen sulfide supplies.

At face value, this might seem disturbing. You see, at least in high concentrations hydrogen sulfide is poisonous or highly dangerous at the very least. To put this into clear focus, hydrogen sulfide is a byproduct of oil refining. The rotten-egg smell is a big tip-off.

Understandably, then, for many generations people have been both confused and somewhat mystified by garlic's supposed dangers and benefits. On the positive side, Mother Nature commands that the human body make its own natural supplies of hydrogen sulfide.

The good news here emerges from the fact that when produced internally within the body hydrogen sulfide acts as an antioxidant. This serves as one of the body's numerous methods of potentially fighting free radicals and cancers while helping to increase blood flow while relaxing blood vessels.

Positive Research Results Emerged

Although the anti-cancer benefits of garlic remain scientifically inconclusive, scientists at the University of Alabama have found a highly promising attribute from this mysterious herb, at least according to one published report.

Researchers at the university discovered that when they introduced small amounts of garlic into human red blood cells, the organisms immediately began producing tiny amounts of hydrogen sulfide.

Certainly much more study is needed. Nonetheless, from my personal view limited numbers of research efforts such as these may indicate that garlic could prove formidable in enabling the body to battle or to prevent prostate, breast and colon cancer.

Perhaps just as important from an overall health prospective, some researchers report that they also believe that garlic might play a critical role in helping to protect the heart.

On the downside, I have never found any undeniable, irrefutable scientific evidence indicating that garlic lowers cholesterol levels.

Even so, at least according to various news articles and published reports, scientists at Albert Einstein College of Medicine discovered that hydrogen sulfide protected the heart muscles of mice that suffered heart attacks.

James W. Forsythe, M.D., H.M.D.

Garlic's Legendary Benefits Prevail

Such positive news regarding garlic hardly comes as a surprise to homeopaths who have known about its strong, positive attributes for many generations. Indeed, as far back as ancient Greece physicians reportedly treated athletes with garlic—sometimes to boost the competitors' strength or endurance before they contributed in Olympic games.

Yet sadly, according to various current published reports, during modern-era the cooking techniques of many chefs inadvertently lessen the positive attributes of garlic. Some chefs unwittingly rob garlic of its beneficial qualities by crushing or chopping it immediately before cooking the herb.

Also on the downside, for the most part the majority of the studies proclaiming garlic as powerful used the equivalent of consuming about two mid-size cloves daily—far more than the average person in the typical U.S. culture ingests.

Such high levels of garlic consumption is typical in numerous other countries where the overall incidence of cancer is lower than in the United States, including South Korea, Italy and specific areas of China.

So, in order to get the formidable anti-cancer benefits of garlic—if, indeed, such attributes exist at all—a typical American would have to drastically increase average daily garlic consumption. Certainly, if the various medical reports are to be believed, eating only one garlic clove per month would do little if anything significant in preventing or controlling cancer.

Embrace Garlic into Your Lifestyle

While the potential strength of garlic in battling cancers remains a matter of dispute, chefs or typical consumers can take some basic easy measures to maximize its benefits.

First, families might consider adding garlic to their typical meal plans on a much more frequent and regular basis.

Also, rather than indiscriminately mashing and overcooking garlic, professional cooks in restaurants and family members should first crush garlic at room temperature before allowing it to sit for at least 15 minutes before cooking begins.

Such tactics are more likely to enable this crop to retain its ability to generate healthful levels of hydrogen sulfide.

All along many consumers likely would remain concerned or at least reluctant to eat this food because it generates specific irritating type of bad breath and perspiration odor that many people consider highly unpleasant or even intolerable. To help neutralize these odors, some consumers might try to use a tactic that has worked effectively for thousands of years in India—eating fennel seeds.

Beware of Outlandish Benefit Claims

The supposed effectiveness of garlic when administered in supplement or pill form remains highly controversial. Within this spectrum, the same warnings and suggestions should apply as listed in the previous chapter on the potential benefits and downsides of vitamin and mineral supplements.

Striving to grab the attention of consumers, some producers of garlic supplements tout their products as being "odorless." Continually mindful of these controversies, some homeopaths and dietitians urge consumers to remember that garlic generally is not considered as a primary food—but rather as beneficial herb used to enhance meal flavors.

Some distributors might claim that garlic can even alleviate high blood pressure or correct hardening of the arteries. The many other attributes supposedly cover everything from diabetes to fever remedies, liver function and even as a treatment for flu or the common cold. Rounding out this diverse mix of ailments that garlic reportedly helps to correct are travelers' diarrhea, osteoporosis and even hay fever.

If all these claims are to be believed, garlic would be the equivalent of the supposed magic, mysterious elixir pitched by unscrupulous medicine hawkers who gained the distinction of being "snake oil salesmen"—particularly in the late 1800s and early 1900s.

Needless to say, today's consumers should remain skeptical regarding such wild one-herb-fixes-all claims. However, during many years as a as a licensed homeopath I've learned that garlic does indeed possess some positive attributes.

Get Professional Guidance

As with all supplements, consumers need to avoid attempts to diagnose themselves or to rush out and buy fad garlic pills online or at their favorite supermarkets.

Consumers should only seek out garlic supplements under the careful supervision of a licensed medical professional who recommends them.

A primary reason for this is the fact that the active ingredient in garlic, the organo-sulfur allicin, changes into various chemical combinations rather quickly when modified. This, in turn, depending on the processing, manufacturing and modification process, could significantly transform the effectiveness of allicin—perhaps eliminating its beneficial properties.

Thus, by striving to generate such attributes as creating "odorless" pills, manufactures may be robbing the garlic of the natural qualities that this herb possesses that make it effective.

Some analysts urge consumers to seek only supplements

that have enteric coating, which strives to enable pills to move relatively undisturbed through the stomach before being absorbed in the intestines. This way the garlic would have a better chance of being fully absorbed into the body, thereby maximizing potential benefits.

Keep an Open Mind

Ultimately, the simple and primary question emerges: "Does garlic actually work in preventing or controlling cancer?"

The overall medical community seems at odds on this issue, some insisting "yes," while others give a resounding "no."

As for my part, I believe that garlic could very well have an essential and helpful place within any anti-cancer diet. While acknowledging that much more research needs to be done, as a medical professional I consider this herb as a formidable potential weapon in assisting the body's fight against the disease.

Nonetheless, I avoid touting garlic as the "magic cure," while also stressing to patients that some physicians might sharply disagree with any proclamation of garlic as being extremely healthful.

In addition, on the rare occasions when I recommend garlic supplements within an individual patient's overall anti-cancer regimen, these referrals come through a certified herbologist—using only products that we deem as potentially effective.

And, finally, patients need to remember that any decision to incorporate garlic into their regular meal plans needs lifelong dedication and unbending commitment.

Chapter 35 Summary

The apparent anti-cancer benefits of garlic remain controversial, with some medical professionals insisting this herb has formidable effectiveness at fighting the disease—while other physicians believe the benefits are miniscule or non-existent. Some studies indicate that the anti-cancer attributes of garlic are extensive, although much more research needs to be done on this issue. The only way to reap benefits from garlic is to eat it on a continuous, non-stop and regular daily basis. To enable garlic to maintain its effective attributes, you should first grind it and then let it sit at least 15 minutes before cooking. The apparent effectiveness of garlic in supplement form remains an issue. Supplement makers that remove odors from garlic during the manufacturing process may be eliminating the herb's effectiveness. Consumers should be cautious about claims that garlic, particularly in supplement form, addresses a wide variety of ailments ranging from the flu to diabetes and heart disease. You should only seek garlic supplements under the guidance of a licensed medical professional. While some physicians claim that garlic has little or no benefits in the fight against and the control of cancer, as an experienced medical professional I personally believe this important herb can serve as a formidable tool in an overall prevention and treatment regimen.

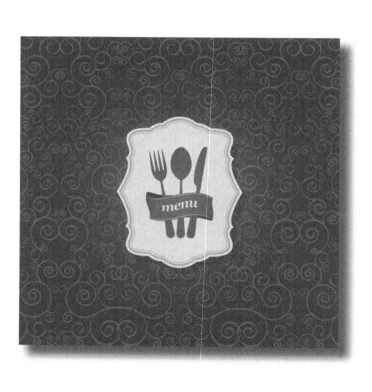

Chapter 36

The Suggested Meal Plan

Please recall amid their recovery regimens, as I've suggested from the start the Forsythe Anti-Cancer Diet does not include a basic, one-plan-fits-all strategy. Depending on their specific medical needs and the objectives set out from my diagnosis, the suggested foods and meal plans will likely vary on a per-patient basis.

Even so, I can list a variety of basic foods that patients should put on their grocery lists for the regular phase of meals after any detoxification (which might not be necessary for every patient.)

Here's the basic grocery list, which might be modified by my clinic staff or dietitians depending on your specific needs:

Protein: Chicken, turkey, any fish (particularly salmon,) extra lean sirloin, flank steak, lean pork and eggs.

Dairy: Only cheese that is feta, 1% cottage cheese, and stony-field plain yogurt.

Nuts: Including butters, these include walnuts, pistachios, pine, pecans, macadamia, filberts, Brazil, cashew and almonds.

Seeds: Including seed butters and pastes, sunflower, pumpkin, sesame and flax.

Mild and mildly starchy vegetables: Asparagus, avocado, green/wax beans, beets and beet greens, bok choy (commonly called "Chinese cabbage," broccoli, Brussels sprouts, cabbage, cauliflower, celery, chard, chicory, collard greens, crookneck squash, cucumber, dandelion, eggplant, endive, escarole, kale, kohlrabi, leek, mustard greens, okra, onion, parsley, parsnips, radishes, romaine lettuce, rutabaga, scallions, spinach, summer squash, Swiss chard, sprouts, turnips, watercress and zucchini.

Starchy vegetables: All colors of peppers, sweet potato, squash, corn and tomato.

Fruits: Apple, apricot, avocado, banana, berries including blackberry, blueberry, huckleberry, raspberry and strawberry, cherimoya, cherries, figs, grapes, grapefruit, kiwi, lemon, limes, loquat, mango, melons including cantaloupe, casaba, Crenshaw, and honeydew, orange, papaya, persimmon, peaches, pear, pineapple, plums, pomegranate, tangerine and tangelos.

Sea Vegetables: Arame, dulse, hijiki, kelp, laver, nori (the Japanese name for edible seaweed,) and wakame.

Grains: Brown rice, barley, oats, quinoa, amaranth and millet.

Oil for salads and cooking: Extra virgin olive oil, sunflower oil, grape seed oil, safflower oil, and coconut oil. (Use flax oil when raw as an essential fatty acid and linolenic acid.) Perhaps flaxseed oil is the best.

Legumes: Adzuki, black-eye peas, black turtle beans, garbanzo beans, kidney beans, lentils, lima beans, mung beans, navy beans, peas, and pinto beans.

In addition, rather than soda, try to use seltzers such as Canada Dry® brand lemon, lime or cherry. Decaf green tea and white tea also make great drinks, especially the Stash® brand.

Meal Plan

Here's my suggested daily meal plan, a recommended cancer protocol for patients who do not yet have a personalized diet from their homeopath or dietitian. (Only use meal schedules such as this after having it reviewed by your medical professional.)

Monday

Breakfast: A two-egg and vegetable omelet with red, green or yellow bell peppers, and spinach, cooked in olive oil or grape seed oil. Eat with decaf green tea and sprouted cereal.

Lunch: Turkey white meat, 2 tablespoons of Dijon® mustard, 1 cup spinach salad, 2 tablespoons of flax oil each with garbanzo beans tossed on the salad.

Dinner: Chicken breast sautéed in grape seed oil, with vegetables such as broccoli, cauliflower and garlic and onion with millet.

Tuesday

Breakfast: Cottage cheese with blueberries and other fresh fruits.

Lunch: Wild rice and black beans, sautéed with onion, garlic and basil, in olive oil with 3 slices of avocado and a salad.

Dinner: Shrimp, broccoli and romaine salad, with oil and vinegar dressing, with any whole grain.

Wednesday

Breakfast: Fresh mozzarella cheese slices and tomato drizzled with olive oil.

Lunch: Salmon and a mixed salad including three slices of avocado, 2 tablespoons of olive oil and vinegar.

Dinner: Turkey breast, 1 cup of cooked asparagus, spinach salad and 2 tablespoons of olive oil.

Thursday

Breakfast: Scrambled eggs with one slice of 100 percent whole Rudolph's rye toast.

Lunch: Chicken salad with 2 tablespoons of olive oil and vinegar dressing.

Dinner: Turkey chili with mixed pinto, kidney or black beans, celery, spices and cayenne pepper.

Friday

Breakfast: A protein shake containing one scoop of 100 percent egg protein such as the brand Healthy 'N Fit® (available at the Vitamin Shoppe™, 1 cup of blueberries, 1 cop of non-sweetened almond milk, 1 tablespoon of flax oil or grounds flax seed meal and ice. People who prefer a thinner shake should add water.

Lunch: Grilled chicken breast with 1 tablespoon of pesto sauce, steamed spinach with rosemary green salad with olive oil, flax oil dressing and quinoa.

Dinner: Turkey breast with broccoli and a mixed green salad containing 2 tablespoons of olive oil and your favorite spice such as basil and oregano.

Saturday

Breakfast: Smoked salmon on rye with crackers.

Lunch: Chicken breast, asparagus or broccoli and one cup of brown rice.

Dinner: Two cups of salad containing romaine, spinach or any of your favorite greens, with 6 ounces of turkey or other protein source, plus olive oil dressing.

Sunday

Breakfast: Plain organic yogurt with an apple or other fruit.

Lunch: Salmon and a spinach salad, olive oil and lemon dressing.

Dinner: Salmon with one half cup of green string beans, mixed greens and olive oil dressing.

Snacks

In addition to the meals listed above, you should enjoy snacks such as nuts, cottage cheese, fruit and other selections from our meal list. Enjoy plain Stony Field yogurt, trail mix, nuts and any type of seeds including dry roasted and low-sodium varieties, granny smith apples with cashew or almond butter, cottage cheese, blueberries with flax oil, protein shakes and leftovers.

Shopping List

- asparagus
- free range eggs
- berries
- brown rice
- almonds
- raw honey
- olive oil
- herbal teas
- brown rice flour
- pumpkin seeds

Chapter 37

Shopping List of Organics

Everyone determined to prevent cancer or to eat better foods amid treatment for the disease, should eat primarily organic foods that have never been processed. Here is a basic list that you can take to the supermarket or to your favorite "natural" or "organic" foods grocery stores:

Vegetables: Artichokes; asparagus, bok choy, broccoli, burdock, cabbage, carrots, celery, chard, corn, diakon-raddish, fennel, garlic, ginger, jicama, kohlrabi, kale, lettuce, mixed green salad, onions, leeks, parsley, potatoes, peas, spinach, squash, string beans, sweet potatoes, tangerine, tomatoes, turnips, winter squash

Fruit: Apples, avocado, bananas, berries, cherries, lemon, oranges, papaya, pear, Satsuma, watermelon

Legumes: Adzuki beans, black beans, chickpeas, kidney beans, lentils, mung beans, white beans

Eggs: Free range

Grains: Amaranth, Basamati rice, brown rice, buckwheat, cornmeal, couscous, millet, polenta, oats (whole and rolled), quinoa, wild rice

Nuts and seeds: Almonds, Brazil nuts, cashews, chia seeds, coconut, flax seeds, hemp seeds, pecans, pumpkin seeds, sesame seeds, sunflower seeds, walnuts

Oils: Coconut oil, ghee, olive oil, sesame oil, toasted sesame oil

Dairy: Living cultures of kefir, yogurt, sour cream, cottage cheese; raw organic milk; raw organic butter; and raw organic cheese

Poultry and seafood: Free range organic poultry; and wild, sustainable harvest fish

Mushrooms: Crimini, miatake, porcini, Portobello, shiitake

Dried herbs and spices: Black pepper, sea salt, cayenne, oregano, basil, thyme, sage

Fresh herbs: Basil, cilantro, Italian flat-leaf parsley, mint

Dried fruits: Apracots, cherries, cranberries, currants, dates, figs, Goji berries, raisins

Condiments: Apple cider vinegar, Balsamic vinegar, Bragg's Amino, gomasio, Mirin, Tamari, brown rice vinegar, Umeboshi vinegar

Canned foods: Coconut milk, chickpeas, black beans, diced tomatoes, tomato sauce, sardines

Beverages: Amazake grain drink, herbal teas, nut milk, oat milk, rice milk

Frozen foods: Corn, berries, peas, spinach

Sea Vegetables: Arame, Dulse flakes, Hijiki, Kombu, Nori, Wakame

Noodles: Asian rice noodles, brown rice pasta, soba noodles, Kamut or spelt pasta, Udon noodles, Quinoa pasta

Flour: Barley flour, brown rice flour, corn meal, spelt flour, garbanzo flour, tapioca flour, quinoa flour and (for those who choose to eat wheat) whole wheat pastry flour

James W. Forsythe, M.D., H.M.D.

Sweeteners: Maple syrup; molasses, raw honey, stevia
Miscellaneous: Bee pollen, green powder, lecithin, mochi, tempeh, whey or rice protein powder.

Chapter 38

Suggested Recipes

Poultry Fun
Chicken With Crusted Herbs

Ingredients

¼ teaspoon black pepper

1 tablespoon butter

2 with tenders removed and each cut crosswise in half, boneless skinless chicken breasts

½ teaspoon salt

¼ cup fresh lemon juice

1 ½ tablespoon minced fresh rosemary

1 tablespoon olive oil

3 tablespoons minced fresh parsley

½ ~ ¾ cup dried bread crumbs (may be freshly ground)

¼ cup lemon juice

Instructions

Prepare: On two separate sheets or wax paper, place each chicken. Pound until ½ inch thick with mallet. Then, with lemon juice toss each chicken until evenly coated. Afterward, cover and refrigerate at least one hour, or even overnight.

Set-up: Pre-heat oven at 450 degrees

Mix: In a small dish melt the olive oil and butter together. (Those wanting to avoid butter can use only olive oil.)

Separate assembly: In a shallow bowl mix the pepper, sea salt, herbs and crumbs.

Chicken: After removing each chicken from the lemon juice, brush the olive oil and butter mixture on both sides (or just the olive oil if no butter is used). Then, put the chicken into a bowl containing herbs and breadcrumbs. Press the herb mixture onto both sides of the chicken.

Cook: On a baking sheet, bake the coated chicken about 12 to 15 minutes until golden brown and cooked through. (Cooking time will depend on the chicken's thickness.)

Suggestion: You can start preparation early, such as preparing break crumb mixture in the morning, or pounding chicken the previous day. Some long-term planners like to double the recipe, enabling them to freeze cooked chicken for later use. Also, butchers can sometimes pound the chicken for consumers who feel weak.

Strength Boosters
Ginger Glycerite

Many cancer patients undergoing various challenging treatments including chemotherapy experience nausea. Many homeopaths and natural-health practitioners believe ginger glycerite helps some of these patients. To maximize the body's absorbtion of fresh ginger, this extraordinary substance is changed into a food-grade glycerin. However, patients should only use this recipe under the specific recommendations and monitoring of a physician, because ginger can possibly thin the blood lower platelet counts.

Ingredients

1 cup food-based vegetable glycerin

¼ pound fresh ginger, preferably organic

Instructions

Prepare: Place the ginger in a food processor after roughly chopping this spice. Keep processing until the liquid is fully mixed.

Change container: Mark pint-size jars with the date and tightly screw the lids after putting in the mixture.

Aging and Shaking: Leave the containers on a counter for at least two weeks, allowing the mixture to macerate. At least every other day or more frequently if you want during this period shake each jar.

Straining: Into a clean jar, strain the mixture through several cheesecloth layers beginning at least two weeks after initially making it.

Refrigeration: This mixture will remain viable for at least six months while jarred without any need for refrigeration.

Suggestion: Some people like to drink ginger glycerite mixed with tea, sparkling water or water. A good starting point is about 1 teaspoon per liquid cup; people who prefer can add more. Patients can drink as often as they prefer for digestive problems or nausea.

Gosamio

This flavor-filled natural treat can be used to replace table salt—thus reducing sodium problems—while also packed with iron, protein, fiber and a little calcium

Basic Ingredients

¼ cup raw organic sesame seeds, any color

1 teaspoon sea salt

1-2 teaspoons dulse or nori flakes or powder. (this is optional)

½ teaspoon dried garlic (optional)

Instructions

Start: After placing the seeds in a heavy-bottom, dry frying pan, you should set the heat at low while stirring often to toast these ingredients. As soon as they start to pop, remove from the stove into a small bowl. Cook as long and as slow as possible to increase flavor intensity. Expect to wait at least 20 minutes for the toasting on a low flame.

Chill: For at least ten minutes cool the seeds. Grind them in a spice grinder with the garlic, dulse and sea salt. Stop when some seeds have cracked. This will have some texture when done properly.

Storage: Keep in a small jar, perfect for use on a variety of foods including steamed vegetables, grains and small salads. This recipe makes about ¼ cup. Store this mixture in the refrigerator if you do not use it within a few weeks.

Stress Reduction Snack

These are designed to help reduce stress, using herbs sometimes deemed as helpful in helping people enhance their emotional well-being.

Basic ingredients

1 cup melted coconut oil

2 cups almonds, soaked for 12 hours, drained and then baked in a 200-degree oven for 2-4 hours

¼ ~ ½ cup honey

1 cup shredded coconut

6 tablespoons eleuthero powder

1/3 cup gourmet mushroom powder

2 tablespoons schisandra berry powder

¼ slippery elm powder

2 tablespoons ashwaganda powder

1 tablespoon licorice powder

2 tablespoons turmeric

¼ cup unsweetened cocoa powder

1 teaspoon vanilla extract

Shredded toast coconut for rolling

Spice Variations

1 tablespoon ground cardamom, ½ teaspoon nutmet and 1 ½ teaspoons ground cinnamon, or

2 teaspoon ground sinnamon, ¾ teaspoon ground nutmeg and ¼ teaspoon ground cloves, or

1 tablespoon ground ginger and 1 teaspoon ground cinnamon

Instructions

Set-up: Process honey, coconut oil and almonds in a food processor until creamy, and then place in a large bowl

Addition: Add vanilla, unsweetened coconut powder, powdered herbs, mushroom powder, coconut or another choice of spices. Mix evenly with hands.

Balls: Use a level tablespoon to roll the mixture into balls. Then roll each ball into shredded coconut

Suggestions: Some health practitioners recommend eating at least one daily.

Nutritional Carrot Congee

Packed with natural nutrients, this porridge has been hailed as often helpful for people who have lost their appetites due to extreme illness. Some homeopaths believe this form of fennel carrot congee, sometimes simplified by cooking just the broth and rice, assists the digestive system.

Ingredients:

5 cups chicken or vegetable stock, or immune or chicken-bone broth

1 carrot, slicked or chopped

1 cup brown or white basmati rice

¼ cup chopped fennel bulb

Instructions

Start: Use a rice cooker or slow cooker filled with vegetables, rice and water.

Prepare: Cook at the lowest possible temperature to cook 4-6 hours. Add enough water to give a soup-like consistency

Suggestions: To boost protein, some people like to add chicken or fish, and ½ cup of leeks, onion or mushrooms can add flavor.

Chicken Bone Broth

This hearty mixture can be helpful in building strength during illness or amid recovery.

Ingredients:

2 juniper or allspice berries

2 bay leaf

1 whole grass-fed organic chicken, cut into quarters or 2-3 pounds of bony chicken parts such as wings, necks and backs

3 stalks celery, chopped

5 quarts cold water

2 carrots, chopped

2 tablespoons apple cider vinegar or lemon juice

1 large onion, chopped

3-inhc piece kombu seaweed (discard after use

Instructions:

Start: Bring chicken and water to a boil in a large pot. Then, simmer for about 1 ½ to 2 hours until meat is tender, easily falling off bones.

Separate: Put meat from the chicken parts and the broth into separate bowls

Cool: Remove the meat from the bones and refrigerate it, and allow chicken to cool.

Resume: Add the vegetables, kombu, lemon juice and apple cider vinegar with the bones and broth into a pot.

Re-Cook: Reduce heat to very low after initially bringing to a boil. On reduced heat cover and simmer 12-24 hours until the marrow is gone from the bones. Cooking slower will result in more nutrients. Add water as needed, checking this level every few hours.

Strain: Strain the broth to remove vegetable matter and bones.

Cool: Place broth into refrigerator after completely cooling. Use a spoon to remove the fat from the top.

Results: Use the chicken for stew or salad, and store the bone broth in the freezer or refrigerator for later use.

Variations: This recipe derived from a variety of sources can include ¼ ounce of dried sliced reishi mushrooms, ½ ounce of astragalus root, or ½ ounce dried codonopsis root.

Broth for Boosting Immunity

This broth is loaded with high-quality organic herbs. To acquire these or to get the best variations, first consult your homeopath or a certified herbologist recommended by that health professional

Ingredients:

2 allspice or juniper berries

3 unpeeled carrots with green tops if possible, cut in thirds

1 medium unpeeled onion, cut into chunks

6 black peppercorns

4 ribs celery, cut into thirds

1 bay leaf

2 cloves garlic, unpeeled

3-inch piece of kombu seaweed (discard after using)

1 large yam or sweet potato cut into chunks

2 red potatoes, quartered

Optional herbs

1 ounce astragalus root slices (about a handful)

½ ounce dried sliced reishi mushrooms (a small handful)

1 ounce dried condonopsis root (about ¼ cup)

Instructions:

Clean: Avoid peeling all vegetables, but wash them

Implement: Use a large pot to hold all ingredients. Cover with from 4 to 4 ½ quarters of water, bringing to a boil

Change: After reaching a boil, reduce heat to low and then partially cover the pot. Simmer as needed 1-4 hours, adding more water as necessary

Cool: Use a fine mesh strainer to strain the stock after allowing broth to cool

Storage: Ideal for storing for up to two months in the freezer or up to one week in the refrigerator. This makes about 3 quarts.

History: This recipe was adapted from a variety of printed sources.

Chilled Energy Balls

Always carry a child-friendly natural source of quick energy, packed with nutritious organic ingredients.

Basic Ingredients

2 cups almond, peanut or sesame peanut butter

3 tablespoons flax, chia or hemp seeds, soaked for 30 minutes and then dried

¼ ~ ½ cup unsweetened cocoa powder

1 tablespoon of almond or vanilla extract

1 cup pitted dates
1 cup dried apples
½ cup dried apricots
½ cup raisins
¼ cup honey (optional)
1-2 tablespoons blackstrap molasses (optional)
¼ goji berries, soaked 30 minutes, then drained
2 tablespoons dried green food supplement
¼ ~ ½ cup juice, tea, or water for smoothness
Pinch of cinnamon or other tasty spice
1 tablespoon nutritional yeast or protein powder (optional)

Rolling Ingredients
2 cups shredded unsweetened, toasted coconut
½ cup sesame seeds or finely ground nuts

Mix: Place the ingredients into a food processor, and process until it is smooth and evenly combined, adding the juice, water or tea as needed to get a firm but roll-able consistency

First roll: Roll into Balls, using about 1 tablespoon of the mixture at a time. You may need to wet your hands slightly to prevent sticking.

Second roll: Roll into balls in shredded coconut, sesame seeds or ground nuts

Chill: Refrigerate in an airtight container with wax or parchment paper between layers, and then chill. This makes about 24 falls.

Non-child friendly: For people who prefer less sweet child-friendly snack, avoid using the unsweetened cocoa powder and the vanilla or almond extract

Fish
Herbed Fish, Moroccan-Style

Ingredients

6-8 small fish steaks or fillets, about 6 ounces each

¼ cup fresh lemon juice

1 large bunch fresh stemmed cilantro

½ cup extra virgin olive oil

1 large bunch fresh stemmed parsley

1 tablespoon sweet paprika

2 tablespoons fresh minced garlic

1 tablespoon ground cumin

1 teaspoon sea salt

Instructions

Break Up: The parsley and cilantro need to be roughly chopped. Then, place them with the garlic in a food processor. Mince, before adding lemon juice, olive oil, sea salt, paprika and cumin. Use the machine again to process.

Prepare: Use a greased baking dish for the fish, and pre-heat oven at 350 degrees.

Side mixture: Warm the herb mixture in a skillet, careful to avoid boiling but until ingredients are hot. Adjust seasoning as needed. Let the fish sit for 15 minutes after spooning the mixture over them.

Cook: Depending on the thickness and type of fish, bake for 10-12 minutes, at least until cooked through.

Roasted Salmon, Rosemary-Style

Ingredients

4-6 salmon fillets

2 lemons, very thinly sliced

2-3 tablespoons olive oil

8-12 springs rosemary
Pepper and sea salt
1 red onion, very thinly sliced
Instructions:
Prepare: After pre-heating the oven at 400 degrees, on a baking sheet arrange rosemary in a single later. Atop the rosemary, cover with red onion slices

Salmon: Put the salmon on top of the onion; sprinkle pepper and sea salt. Place lemon slices atop the salmon. Drizzle this with olive oil.

Cook: Roast 12-18 minutes in pre-heated oven, until when salmon is cooked through. This serves four to six people.

Vegetarian Dishes
Mushroom and Asparagus Quiche

Ingredients
1 whole grain or spelt pie crust
2 ounces grated gruyere cheese
1 tablespoon olive oil
2 tablespoons chopped fresh dill
¾ tablespoon sea salt, divided into thirds
¼ teaspoon sea salt
1 ½ cups asparagus, tough ends discarded, sliced into 1-inch lengths
½ cup half and half, or cream
1 cup shiitake or cremini mushrooms, thinly sliced with stems cut off
1 cup milk
1 teaspoon minced garlic
3 large eggs
Instructions:

Prepare: After preheating the oven at 375 degrees, sauté the asparagus about 5-6 minutes until just tender in olive oil with ¼ teaspoon of sea salt. Set aside inside a bowl after being careful to avoid overcooking. In the same pan, sauté the mushrooms until tender with ¼ teaspoon of sea salt. Sauté for another 30 seconds with garlic. Set aside after tossing the asparagus with mushrooms.

Mix: Whisk the fresh herbs, sea salt, milk, half and half and eggs in a large bowl.

Shell: Sprinkle grated cheese atop the bottom of the pie shell. Evenly place mushroom and asparagus mixture over the cheese.

Pour: Up to the rim of the pie shell, put the egg mixture over the vegetables.

Cook: Bake until the custard mixture is completely set, usually about 40-50 minutes. Cool slightly before cutting. Recipe makes 4-6 servings.

Suggestions: As a time saver, you can grate the cheese the previous day, and prepare the vegetables two days early. For variety, this recipe has numerous variations. You might try ½ to 1 cup of grated cheese, or from ½ to ¾ cup of feta or goat cheese. Consider sprinkling cheese on all the various layers. Some chefs prefer using 1 ½ to 2 cups of sliced turkey bacon, diced sausage or chicken, shrimp, or cooked vegetables, or flaked salmon.

Vegetable Lasagna

Ingredients

8 ounces grated mozzarella cheese

2 (24-ounce) jars organic pasta sauce of any flavor, or 6 cups of homemade sauce

1 pound lasagna noodles (prefer rice or whole grain)

½ teaspoon dried oregano

2 tablespoons olive oil

½ teaspoon sea salt

1 small yellow onion, about 1 ½ cups finely chopped

2 orange, yellow or red bell peppers, diced and seeded

2 tablespoons minced garlic

1 chopped zucchini

2 (10-ounce) packages chopped frozen spinach, drained well and thawed, or 4 bunches fresh spinach, cleaned, cooked just to wilt and then pressed to remove water and divided into two portions

4 cups part-skim ricotta cheese

1 teaspoon black pepper

1 large egg

¼ cup Parmesan cheese

Instructions

Cook: After bringing to a boil a large pot of salted water, add lasagna noodles and cook.

Mix: Stir a couple times in the beginning to prevent noodles from sticking together.

Remove: Drain and rinse in cold water immediately after the noodles reach "al dente." (See the package for details) Then, set the separated noodles aside.

Addition: Mix the pepper, sea salt, Parmesan, egg and ricotta. Add half of the spinach mix to combine evenly, and then set aside.

Suggestions: Many tasks can be done well ahead of time, such as grating cheese up to 2 days early, or preparing vegetables a few days beforehand.

Extraordinary Pasta

Ingredients

½ cup crumbled feta, blue cheese, fresh grated Parmesan cheese, or Gorgonzola cheese (this is optional)

2 tablespoons olive oil

½ cup chopped parsley

2 medium onions, thinly sliced and cut in half

12 ounces kamut or other whole grain pasta

1 tablespoon garlic

¼ cup sun-dried tomatoes in oil, chopped (optional)

4 cups butternut squash, or peeled and diced delicate

2 bunches chard, stems removed, washed and chopped, or use collard greens or kale

Instructions

Prepare: First use a large skillet to heat olive oil at medium. Stir often while adding and cooking onions. Continue 15-20 minutes until they're golden brown

More: Add diced winter squash and garlic. Then, reduce heat slightly, cover the pan and cook about 5 minutes

Complete: Add sun-dried tomatoes and chard, before covering and continuing to cook for about 10 minutes until all vegetables become tender. Avoid worrying if ingredients start sticking. If this happens add about ¼ cup of water to the pan

Separate pot: As the vegetables cook, bring to a boil a large pot of sea-salted water. Follow package directions in cooking pasta until this becomes "al dente." At that point, drain, mix under hot water and return to the pot.

Perfection: Toss the vegetables when they become tender, combining with the chopped fresh parsley and the pasta. Afterward, if desired garnish this with cheese. Recipe makes 4-6 servings

Suggestions: Some chefs like to add cubed cooked chicken or cooked and sliced chicken sausage. Early preparation can include cooking pasta the previous night or in the morning, or getting vegetables ready up to two days early.

Healthy Salads
Fruity Salad with Quinoa

Ingredients

2 tablespoons minced fresh cilantro

1 cup quinoa, soaked overnight, then rinsed well in a mesh colander

2 tablespoons soaked, dehydrated toasted almonds

½ tablespoon mirin

¼ to ½ cup red onion, finely diced

2 teaspoons grated fresh ginger

1 tablespoon golden or regular raisins

1 tablespoon dried goji berries

1/3 cup dried apricots, diced

¼ teaspoon sea salt

1 tablespoon olive oil

½ cup orange juice

¾ cup water

Instructions

Boiling: Bring water to boil, along with sea salt, olive oil, orange juice.

Mix: Add ginger, dried fruit and quinoa to the boiling mixture, then cover reducing heat to low for 10-15 minutes, or quinoa becomes tender and all water is absorbed. Afterward, let ingredients sit covered 15 minutes

Separate: After bringing water to a boil in a separate small pot, add diced red onion for 15 seconds and then drain well. To bring out the pink color, toss with mirin.

Bowl: Turn the quinoa when tender in a bowl. Using fork, gently fluff together with toasted almonds and onions. Those who prefer can garnish with a bit of cilantro. This makes 2-3 servings, best served at room temperature or warm.

Suggestions: Preparation is easy, so little if any early preparation is necessary—although topping apricots, red onion and toasted almonds can be done up to a day early.

Arugula, Barley and Beet Salad
Ingredients
1 pound beets, trimmed and separated
4 cups water
1 small piece kombu seaweed (discard after use)
Dressing ingredients
1 (4-ounce package) crumbled feta cheese or goat cheese (optional)
1 bunch arugula, washed and roughly chopped, about 4-5 cups
¼ cup walmuts or pecans, toasted
½ teaspoon sea salt
¼ cup balsamic vinegar
2 tablespoons olive oil
2 teaspoons fennel seeds, toasted and crushed or roughly chopped
½ teaspoon sea salt
Instructions
Start: Cover the beets with water in a saucepan and bring to boil. Then, depending on the size and age of the beets, simmer 15-20 minutes partly covered until beets are tender when poked with fork. Afterward, drain and rinse under cold water after they have become tender. Wait until the skins are cool enough to handle, and then slip off the skins and slice beets into wedges before setting

them aside.

Side preparation: In a separate pot while beets cook, bring kombu, water and barley to a boil. Reduce head to low, cover and cook 20-25 minutes or until barley is tender. Drain, rinse under cold water and drain again. Discard the kombu, and place the barley in a large bowl.

Mix: Whisk together the sea salt, fennel seeds, olive oil and balsamic vinegar. Toss the dressing with the barley before adding arugula, toasted walnuts and beets, and cheese if desired. Toss gently to combine. Recipe makes about 2 quarts of salad.

Time saver: You can cook the beets and barley, and the dressing, a day early.

Toasted Cashews with Millet and Broccoli
Ingredients
¼ cup minced fresh parsley
¼ cup minced fresh dill weed
1 cup cherry tomatoes, sliced in half
1 cup millet, soaked overnight
2 cups boiling water
¼ teaspoon sea salt
2 cups broccoli, florets and chopped stems
¾ cup thinly sliced celery
Dressing Ingredients
½ teaspoon sea salt
½ - 1 cup cashews, toasted
1 teaspoon minced garlic
1/3 cup olive oil
1/3 cup fresh lemon juice
Instructions
Start: In a saucepan over medium heat, toast the millet stirring

constantly until gives off a nutty fragrance and begins to turn brown

Addition: Carefully add the boiling water and sea salt, reduce the heat to low and cover. Cook about 20-25 minutes until the water is absorbed and the millet is tender.

Cooling: Spread the millet out on a cookie sheet to cool

Continue: While millet cools, steam broccoli just until tender and bright green Rinse under cold water, drain well and place in a large bowl. Then, add the parsley, dill, tomatoes and celery to the broccoli.

Mix: Whisk the lemon juice, sea salt, garlic and olive oil in a separate bowl. When the millet is cool, crumble it into the vegetables. Add the dressing and cashews, tossing everything together. Recipe makes 7-8 cups.

Suggestions: Salad usually tastes best on the day it's prepared. For variation, consider using different grains such as bulgur wheat, quinoa or millet. As a time saver, all vegetables can be washed and chopped up to two days early.

Aduki Bean and Millet Salad
Lemon cumin dressing ingredients
Fresh ground pepper to taste
½ teaspoon sea salt
4 tablespoons olive oil
Zest of one lemon
4 tablespoons fresh lemon juice
½ teaspoon ground cumin
Salad ingredients
1 cup millet, soaked overnight
2 cups boiling water
Pinch sea salt

½ cup fresh parsley, chopped

2 cups cooked aduki beans or (14-ounce) can aduki beans, drained and rinsed

½ cup red onion, diced and sautéed briefly

1 pint cherry tomatoes, cut in half

1 cup fresh corn, cut from the cob and sautéed for 1-2 minutes, or frozen corn thawed, or 1 cup peeled, seeded and diced cucumber

Instructions

Prepare: While stirring constantly over medium heat, toast the millet in a saucepan. Do this until millet gives off a nutty fragrance and begins to turn brown.

Addition: Carefully add sea salt and boiling water, reducing heat and covering. Then, cook 20-25 minutes until millet is tender and water is absorbed.

Cool: Spread millet onto cookie sheet to cool.

Continue: While millet cools, whisk together pepper, sea salt, cumin, lemon zest and juice and olive oil for the dressing. Then, prepare the remaining ingredients.

Tossing: In a bowl after millet is cool crumble it and toss with dressing. Toss again upon adding all remaining ingredients, mixing evenly. Recipe makes about 6 cups.

Time saver: Dressing, millet and beans can be made or prepared a day early.

Rice Noodle Salad

Ingredients

4 ounces Asian rice noodles (makes about 3 ½ cups cooked noodles)

Dressing Ingredients

1-2 teaspoons minced ginger

1 tablespoon maple syrup

2 tablespoons toasted sesame oil

2 tablespoons tamari or Bragg's Aminos

1 ½ tablespoon rice vinegar

Optional ingredients

Whole cilantro leaves or thinly sliced scallions

2-4 tablespoons toasted sesame seeds, cashews or peanuts

4-8 ounces shrimp, tempeh or chicken

2-4 cups steamed, sautéed or raw vegetables of choice

Instructions

Mix: Whisk together basic listed primary dressing ingredients

Cook: Bring large pot of water to a boil before adding noodles. For 3-4 minutes until noodles finish cooking, continuously use fork or tongs to pull apart strands to prevent them from sticking. Drain noodles and mix well as soon as they taste tender.

Toss: Mix about half the dressing with the noodles. Then, add any other proteins or vegetables that you want along with enough dressing to flavor and moisten mixture.

Garnish: Use nuts, sliced scallions, cilantro leaves or sesame seeds to garnish as desired. Recipe makes 3 ½ - 5 cups, depending on what is added.

Time saver: You can make dressing up to 1 week early before refrigerating prior to use. Prepare vegetables up to two days early.

Suggestions: Consider limitless possibilities for variation, everything from sautéed shiitake mushrooms to steamed broccoli florets, or cooked chicken or shrimp. For added nutrition, add from ½ to 1 cup each of two to four vegetables.

Herb Marinated Vegetables Salad

Ingredients

6 cups whole Yukon gold potatoes, scrubbed and then boiled until tender

¼ - ½ red onion, sliced thinly

¼ cup fresh dill, chopped

¼ cup fresh basil, chopped

½ cup fresh parsley, chopped

½ cup Kalamata or Nicoise olives, pitted and halved

1 cup cheery tomatoes, halved, or 1 small red bell pepper, diced or sliced and sautéed briefly

6 ounces marinated artichoke hearts, drained and sliced

Red wine vinaigrette ingredients

2 tablespoons capers, drained and minced

3 tablespoons red wine vinegar

Zest and juice of one lemon

1 tablespoon Dijon mustard

¼ teaspoon each sea sale and pepper, or to taste

8-9 tablespoons olive oil

Instructions

Multi-task: As potatoes cook, whisk together lemon juice, vinegar, and red wine, and zest Dijon, sea salt, olive oil, capers, and pepper and set aside

Prepare: Rinse the potatoes in cold water when tender, drain and then refrigerate. When the potatoes become cool enough to handle, dice them or cut into wedges, before tossing them with a small amount of the dressing.

Addition: Along with any additional steamed vegetables that you want, mix the rest of the ingredients with as much dressing as desired. Toss evenly. Recipe makes 6-8 cups.

Suggestions: Various types of vegetables are optional, including: cauliflower or broccoli florets, steamed until tender; asparagus trimmed and cut into 1-inch lengths and steamed until crisp tender; and green beans, trimmed and cut into 1-inch lengths, steamed until crisp and tender.

Wild Rice Salad

Ingredients

1 ¼ cup brown basmati rice, soaked overnight
½ cup wild rice, soaked overnight
1 tablespoon hone or maple syrup
1 teaspoon sea salt
1/3 cup lemon juice
1/3 cup olive oil
1 cup cooked garbanzo beans (optional)
1 bunch scallions, thinly sliced and trimmed
1 ½ cups red and / or green grapes, cut in half
¾ cup minced fresh parsley
1 cup toasted walnuts or toasted pecans

Instructions

Cook: First, drain the brown rice and place with ¼ teaspoon sea salt and 1 ¾ cups water in a small saucepan. Initially bring to a boil, and then reduce to low, cover and cook 25-30 minutes until tender and all water is absorbed. Afterward, cook rice in large bowl.

Separate: Bring the rice to an initial boil in 2 cups of water in another saucepan, before simmering on low 30-35 minutes heat until tender. Drain wild rice and add to the brown rice.

Mix: Whisk the sweetener, sea salt, lemon juice and olive oil until the dressing thickens.

Toss: After the rice cools, toss and coat with dressing. Then, add the remaining ingredients before tossing again. Recipe makes 7-8 cups.

Time saver: You can whisk dressing ingredients up to a week early, and cook the rice a day beforehand.

Suggestion: For added protein, consider adding tempeh, turkey or chicken.

Healthy Breakfasts
Applesauce Muffins

Ingredients

1 cup pecans, almonds or chopped walnuts

½ cup goji berries, raisins, dried cranberries or currants

1 ½ cup whole wheat pastry flour or brown rice, oat, barley or quinoa flour

½ cup molasses, or ¼ cup molasses and ¼ cup maple syrup or another sweetener

1 cup applesauce

¼ cup melted coconut oil

Pinc ground cloves

½ teaspoon sea salt

½ teaspoon baking soda

¾ teaspoon cinnamon

1 ½ teaspoon non-aluminum baking powder

Instructions

Prepare: Flour and grease a 12-cup muffin tin, and pre-heat oven at 350 degrees

Mix: Shift dry ingredients together. Also, whisk the molasses, applesauce and oil in a separate bowl

Add: Combine and stir the dry and liquid ingredients. Then, add the nuts and dried fruits, stirring evenly to combine.

Insert: Put the batter into the muffin tins

Cook: Cook until inserting a toothpick into the center exits clean, usually about 20 minutes. This recipe makes 12 muffins.

Time saver: Mixing of wet and dry ingredients can be done a day early.

Suggestion: Store a batch in your freezer inside a zipped bag.

Breakfast Pudding

Ingredients

1 cup amaranth

Who dairy milk or non-dairy alternative

3 cups water or half water and half dairy or non-dairy milk

¼ cup almonds, toasted and chopped

¼ cup dried cherries

1-2 tablespoons honey or maple syrup

1 teaspoon vanilla extract

½ cup goji berries

¼ teaspoon ground nutmeg

½ teaspoon ground coriander

½ teaspoon ground cinnamon

6 dates, shopped

Instructions:

Cooking: After combining water and the amaranth in a medium saucepan, initially bring to boil before reducing heat to low. Cover pot after adding dried fruit, and then cooking until creamy for about 20 minutes.

Mix: Stir in the chopped almonds, ground spices, vanilla, and sweetener if you're using it. Then, stir in the milk if desired before serving. Recipe serves four

Suggestion: Besides for a breakfast, this recipe also can be used for a dessert.

Healthy Desserts
Poaching Fruit

Since most fruits, especially citrus, are antioxidants they can serve as tasty, slightly sweet desert-like treats—especially when properly prepared.

Ingredients

¼ cup dried cherries

2 dried figs, quartered

1 ½ cups water

4 apples, quartered, peeled and cored

4 pears, ripe but firm, quartered, peeled and cored

2 two-inch cinnamon sticks

¼ ~ ½ cup organic maple syrup

Zest of 1 orange

Instructions

Combine: Mix ingredients

Cook: Simmer in a large pot

Add: pears and apples

Simmer: Slowly cook for about 10 minutes

More: When the fruit is barely tender, add dried fruit. Then, cook for about 10 minutes until the fruit is tender and fruit is reduced by half.

Suggestions: You can serve this warm or chilled, always a tasty, low-calorie snack—particularly a good energy booster when eaten two or three hours after main meals.

Baked Apples

For added zip, on the day before preparing the primary recipe, you can zest oranges, dates and goji berries.

Ingredients

¼ teaspoon ground cloves

¼ teaspoon ground ginger

½ ground cardamom

1 teaspoon ground cinnamon

½ cup oat flakes or quinoa

3 teaspoons butter or coconut oil

½ cup almonds, toasted and chopped

1 orange, zested and juiced

4 dates, chopped

2 tablespoons goji berries

6 large apples

Instructions

Prepare: Put apples on a 9-inch by 13-inch greased baking dish, and set the oven at 350 degrees

Main fruits: Zest and juice the orange rind before juicing it. Use this to soak the dates and goji berries.

Combine: Mix all the spices, butter or oil, almonds, and oat flakes or quinoa. Then, combine thoroughly with the goji berry mixture.

Fruit containers: Put this mixture into the apples

Cook: For 35 minutes to 45 minutes, bake the apples until tender under foil.

Upside-down Pie

Homeopaths like this recipe partly because the mixture has no added white sugars. A great snack for any time, upside-down pies can be particularly yummy when pears and sweet potatoes serve as the primary ingredients. As a time-saving measure, you can prepare the crust and start storing it a few days in advance of baking.

Almond Top Crust Ingredients

1 teaspoon vanilla extract

½ cup melted coconut oil and ghee

3 tablespoons apple or orange juice

2 cups almonds, finely ground in food processor

¼ cup wheat, spelt or rice flour

2 rolled oats or quinoa flakes

1 tablespoon ground cinnamon

Filling Ingredients

1 tablespoon tapioca flour, arrowroot or cornstarch

¼ teaspoon sea salt

4 pears, cored and sliced about ¼-inch thick

¾ cup apple cider, or orange or apple juice

2 medium sweet potatoes, peeled and sliced into ¼-inch thick rounds

¼ cup goji berries

1 tablespoon fresh lemon juice

Instructions

Prepare: Grease a 13-inch by 9-inch baking dish, and preheat oven at 375 degrees

Combine: Into a large bowl, mix all filling ingredients. Gently toss to evenly coat everything. Spread the filling into the dish.

More mixing: Spread these combined ingredients evenly atop the filling, after mixing all these items in a separate bowl.

Cook: Bake until topping becomes golden and crisp and the filling is soft, usually 45-60 minutes.

Dairy-Free Treats

Perfect for anyone who craves sweetness, when prepared correctly this has the texture of soft ice cream. Here are two-frequently used recipes:

Banana Coconut

Ingredients

1-2 tablespoons honey or maple syrup (optional)

5 bananas, peeled and frozen

1 teaspoon vanilla extract

One 15-ounce can of coconut milk

¼ cup coconut cream or coconut flakes

Instructions

Blend: Mix all ingredients until creamy and smooth in a blender, except the bananas. Then, use ice cube trays for freezing this mixture.

Wait: Allow the coconut to soften, and after the mixture freezes remove before processing.

Juicing: Process the cubes and bananas in a juicer, setting the machine so that the mixture becomes a puree.

Option: Rather than processing the bananas along with the cubes in a juicer as above, instead break up the frozen banana and process with slightly softened coconut cubes in a food processor.

Apple or Pear Ginger Crisp

Although a healthy desert, this can serve as an excellent treat at any time of day, even for breakfast.

Oat Topping Ingredients

1 teaspoon almond extract

2 cups rolled oats

1/4 to ½ cup maple syrup or honey

1 cup whole wheat, spelt or rice flour

1/3 cup almond or walnut oil

1 cup almonds, toasted or chopped

Pinch of sea salt

Filling Ingredients

1 tablespoon arrowroot, corn starch or tapioca flour

8 large pears or apples

¼ cup maple syrup or honey

½ cup apple juice or cider

1 teaspoon almond extract

Zest of one orange

2 teaspoons freshly grated or minced ginger

Instructions

Prepare: Place the apples or pears—sliced, cored and peeled—into a greased 9-inch by 13-inch pan or casserole dish. Set the oven at 350 degrees

Mix: Combine the apple juice, orange zest, ginger, syrup, and almond extract into a bowl. Then whisk in the arrowroot until the mixture becomes smooth. Pour this onto the fruit and set aside.

Separate combination: Mix the pinch of sea salt, flour, almonds and oats into a separate bowl. Then whisk the almond extract, oil and syrup separately before tossing and combining this liquid with the oat mixture.

Zest: Sprinkle the oat topping over the apples pears or apples, before baking 35 minutes under foil. Then, remove the foil before baking an additional 15 minutes as the fruit gets tender and the top becomes browned.

Recommended Reading

A variety of publications provide helpful information on anti-cancer recipes. Among those worth reviewing:

"The Cancer-Fighting Kitchen," Rebecca Katz, Random House, 2009

"Cooking With Foods That Fight Cancer," Richard Beliveau, Denis Gingras, McClelland & Stewart, 2007

"One Bite at a Time, Nourishing Recipes for Cancer Survivors and Their Friends," Rebecca Katz, Celestial Arts Press, 2008

"The What to Eat if you Have Cancer Cookbook (Revised): Healing Foods that Boost Your Immune System," Daniella Chace and Maureen Keane, McGraw Hill, 2006

Herbal Information

"Adaptogens: Herbs for Strength, Stamina & Stress Relief," David Winston and Steven Maimes, Healing Arts Press, 2007

"Breast Cancer? Breast Health! The Wise Woman Way," Susan Weed, Ash Tree Publishing, 1996

"Herbal Medicine, Healing & Cancer," Donald Yance, Keats Publishing, 1999

"Holistic Herbal: A Safe and Practical Guide to Making and Using Herbal Remedies, David Hoffman, 2003

James W. Forsythe, M.D., H.M.D.

About the Author

James W. Forsythe, M.D., H.M.D., has long been considered one of the most respected physicians in the United States, particularly for his treatment of cancer and the legal use of human growth hormone. In the early 1960s, Dr. Forsythe graduated with honors from University California at Berkeley and earned his Medical Degree from University of California, San Francisco, before spending two years residency in Pathology at Tripler Army Hospital, Honolulu. After a tour of duty in Vietnam, he returned to San Francisco and completed an internal medicine residency and an oncology fellowship. He is also a world-renowned speaker and author. He has co-authored, been mentioned in and/or written chapters in bestsellers. To name a few: "An Alternative Medicine Definitive Guide to Cancer;" "KNOCKOUT, Interviews with Doctors who are Curing Cancer" Suzanne Somers' number-one bestseller; "The Ultimate Guide To Natural Health, Quick Reference A-Z Directory of Natural Remedies for Diseases and Ailments;" "Anti-Aging Cures;" "The Healing Power of Sleep;" "Outsmart Your Cancer: Alternative Non-Toxic Treatments That Work and Alternative Medicine Guide 2 Women's Health Series" and "Compassionate Oncology ~ What Conventional Cancer Specialists Don't Want You To Know;" and "Obaminable Care," "Complete Pain," "Natural Pin Killers," and "Your Secret to the Fountain of Youth ~ What They Don't Want You to Know About HGH Human Growth Hormone."

Made in the USA
San Bernardino, CA
28 February 2020

65136203R00239